T0076516

The Underactive Thyroid

Do it yourself because your doctor won't

Dr Sarah Myhill MB BS (HONS)
and
Craig Robinson MA (OXON)

Hammersmith Health Books
London, UK

First published in 2023 by Hammersmith Health Books
– an imprint of Hammersmith Books Limited
4/4A Bloomsbury Square, London WC1A 2RP, UK
www.hammersmithbooks.co.uk

© 2023, Dr Sarah Myhill and Craig Robinson

All rights reserved. No part of this publication may be reproduced, stored in any retrieval system or transmitted in any form or by any means, electronic, mechanical, photocopying, recording or otherwise, without the prior permission of the publishers and copyright holders.

The information contained in this book is for educational purposes only. It is the result of the study and the experience of the authors. Whilst the information and advice offered are believed to be true and accurate at the time of going to press, neither the authors nor the publisher can accept any legal responsibility or liability for any errors or omissions that may have been made or for any adverse effects which may occur as a result of following the recommendations given herein. Always consult a qualified medical practitioner if you have any concerns regarding your health.

British Library Cataloguing in Publication Data: A CIP record of this book is available from the British Library.

Print ISBN 978-1-78161-235-4
Ebook ISBN 978-1-78161-236-1

Commissioning editor: Georgina Bentliff
Designed and typeset by: Julie Bennett of Bespoke Publishing Limited
Cover illustrations: Tashat at Shutterstock
Cover design by: Madeline Meckiffe
Index: Dr Laurence Errington
Production: Deborah Wehner of Moatvale Press, UK
Printed and bound by: TJ Books Limited, Cornwall, UK'

Contents

About the Authors

Dr Sarah Myhill MB BS qualified in medicine (with Honours) from Middlesex Hospital Medical School in 1981 and has since focused tirelessly on identifying and treating the underlying causes of health problems, especially the 'diseases of civilisation' with which we are beset in the West. She has worked in the NHS and private practice and for 17 years was the Honorary Secretary of the British Society for Ecological Medicine, which focuses on the causes of disease and treating through diet, supplements and avoiding toxic stress. She helps to run and lectures at the Society's training courses and also lectures regularly on organophosphate poisoning, the problems of silicone, and chronic fatigue syndrome. Visit her website at www.drmyhill.co.uk

Craig Robinson MA took a first in Mathematics at Oxford University in 1985. He then joined Price Waterhouse and qualified as a Chartered Accountant in 1988, after which he worked as a lecturer in the private sector, and also in the City of London, primarily in Financial Sector Regulation roles. Craig first met Sarah in 2001, as a patient for the treatment of his ME, and since then they have developed a professional working relationship, where he helps with the maintenance of www.drmyhill.co.uk, the moderating of Dr Myhill's Facebook groups and other ad hoc projects, as well as with the editing and writing of her books.

Stylistic note: Use of the first person singular in this book refers to me, Dr Sarah Myhill. One can assume that the medicine and biochemistry are mine, as edited by Craig Robinson and that the classical and mathematical references are Craig's.

Dedication

SM: To Dr Gordon Skinner, Consultant Virologist and pioneer in the treatment of the underactive thyroid. He was hounded to his death by the General Medical Council because he dared to prescribe natural desiccated thyroid to patients who were clinically hypothyroid despite 'normal' blood tests. The fact that he restored the health of thousands of people was of no interest to the medical establishment.

CR: For Louise, my hairdresser, friend and an all-round lovely human being. Louise first started cutting my hair around 25 years ago, when I was very ill with ME, and bedridden. She would come into my bedroom, and I would roll from side to side while she leant over and half-sat on the bed to cut my hair. This simple act made me feel human. Years later I asked her whether she was at all nervous about coming into a strange man's bedroom to which she replied, in typical fashion: 'You were the one who should have been worried – I had the scissors!'

Preface

According to the capabilities of the reader, books have their own destiny.
Robert Burton (8 February 1577 – 25 January 1640),
English writer and fellow of Oxford University,
best known for his encyclopaedic book *The Anatomy of Melancholy*[1]

If what Robert Burton said is true, then it would seem that the destiny of this book is in safe hands. The fact that you are here, dear reader, taking charge of your own health, with an enquiring mind, is good news for you, and also, if Burton is to be believed, good news for this book.

Though the chapter titles in the Contents list for this book are mostly clear, we give readers a bit more detail here about what to expect in each:

- Introduction: Do it yourself because your doctor won't – this describes why this book is necessary and introduces the thyroid gland
- Part I: The practical – provides the Tools of the Trade for looking after your thyroid health, including:
  - Chapter 1: Are you hypothyroid? Poor energy delivery symptoms and signs (including chronic fatigue syndrome, myxoedema madness* and poor

---

* **Historical note on 'Myxoedema madness':** The Committee on Myxoedema of the Clinical Society of London issued the first report (1886) that described the development of 'delusions and hallucinations' in almost half of hypothyroid patients.[2] Sixty years later, in 1949, Asher et al re-examined this relationship in 14 patients who had psychosis and clinical evidence of hypothyroidism. The patients received thyroid hormone supplements, with nine patients achieving full recovery.[3] Asher labelled this association 'myxoedema madness', which later was renamed 'myxoedema psychosis' (MP).

immunity); thyroid-specific symptoms (metabolic, sleep, oedema, skin, hair and nails, bones, constipation, 'signs' (pulse, blood pressure and core temperature)); other clues (family history, other autoimmune conditions, gradual decline); and triggers.

- ○ Chapter 2: Blood tests for underactive thyroid – The stengths and weaknesses of such and what other information is needed.
- ○ Chapter 3: Before you start a trial of thyroid glandular (natural desiccated thyroid) – All the other interventions, especially diet and supplements, that need to be in place before you try out natural thyroid supplementation.
- ○ Chapter 4: The adrenal gearbox – Symptoms, diagnosis and management of adrenal fatigue.
- ○ Chapter 5: How to trial thyroid glandular (natural desiccated thyroid) – Starting low, building slowly and finding your personal 'sweet spot'.
- Part II: The theory – provides the motivation for looking after your thyroid yourself:
  - ○ Chapter 6: How and why we become hypothyroid – The possible causes of primary and secondary hypothyroidism, including autoimmunity, environmental factors and nutritional deficiencies.
  - ○ Chapter 7: What happens if the diagnosis of hypothyroidism is missed – This chapter is a bit scary, itemising accelerated ageing and degeneration, dementia, heart disease and cancer, so it ends with some light relief!
  - ○ Chapter 8: Thyroid myths – This arms you to face discouragement from health professionals about taking charge of your thyroid yourself.
  - ○ Chapter 9: How we starve, destroy and poison the the thyroid – Helps understanding of the ways in which modern life damages the thyroid and how we can limit that damage.
  - ○ Chapter 10: The hypothyroid child – Another scary chapter detailing the consequences for growth and development of mother (during pregnancy) and child being hypothyroid.
  - ○ Chapter 11: The hypothyroid female – Underactive thyroid is much more common in those with female hormones; this chapter explains why and what particular action to take.
  - ○ Chapter 12: Thyrotoxicosis – Addresses the much rarer issue of overactive thyroid and possible causes.
  - ○ Chapter 13: Iodine – How much iodine is it desirable and safe to supplement and

what other uses does iodine have in the body?
- Appendices – including how to access tests, different natural thyroid preparations, and the 'Groundhog regimes' (so-called because we repeat them over and over again – they are so important).

Much of the Appendices is repeated from our other books, though with a particular focus on the underactive thyroid, so that this book can be self-contained and provide all you need. That said, readers will find references to our other books for more detail on the why and how of the paleo-ketogenic diet, understanding and fighting infection, pregnancy and child development, and a comprehensive picture of ecological medicine, including numerous case histories.

Returning to Robert Burton and his tome *The Anatomy of Melancholy*, this, had the original title *The Anatomy of Melancholy, What it is: With all the Kinds, Causes, Symptomes, Prognostickes, and Several Cures of it. In Three Maine Partitions with their several Sections, Members, and Subsections. Philosophically, Medicinally, Historically, Opened and Cut Up.*(By the way, this is not the longest book title ever – that 'honour' belongs to *The Historical Development of the Heart from Its Formation From* ... In all, the title contains 3777 words and over 26,000 characters. But we [Craig!] digress(es).) The title was long, but the thrust of what Burton suggested can easily be distilled down to:
- Diet rectified
- Sleep and waking rectified
- Exercise rectified
- Air rectified
- Mirth, music and merrymaking.

The reader will notice, in due course, that these principles are very similar to the Groundhog regimes described in the Appendices, but do not hurry there yet – there is much reading to be done first!

Introduction

Do it yourself because your doctor won't

My experience, flowing from four decades of clinical medicine and consultations with thousands of patients, has shown me that the best person to effect a cure is the sufferer. No-one is better motivated or better positioned to put in place the interventions which allow healing and recovery. This will not happen with conventional Western medicine because patients have been disempowered by doctors. They believe in pills for all ills. But most physicians and pharmacists are more interested in profits than patients. Big Pharma's mantra is 'A patient cured is a customer lost'.

My job as a physician is to supply the Rules of the Game and the Tools of the Trade to allow patients to find their own path to recovery. From the symptoms, signs and tests, we – the patient and me – together establish the underlying mechanisms which, if uncorrected, progress to pathological disease. This is proper, scientific, logical medicine which goes under various names: naturopathic, ecological, functional. This is not an alternative medicine – it is the Real McCoy.*

*There are many contenders as to the derivation of the phrase 'the real McCoy'. Here are four:
1. Perhaps the McCoy is derived from Mackay, referring to Messrs Mackay of Edinburgh, who distilled a fine whisky from 1856 onwards and who, from 1870, promoted it as 'the real MacKay'
2. The expression could have derived from the name of the branch of the MacKay family from Reay, Scotland, that is, 'the Reay Mackay'.
3. Perhaps it was the Kid McCoy (Norman Selby, 1872-1940), American welterweight boxing champion, who gave us this phrase. The story goes that a drunk challenged Selby to a fight to prove that he was McCoy and not one of the many lesser boxers trading under the same name. After being knocked down, the drunk mumbled, 'Yes, that's the real McCoy'.
4. Or maybe it was named after one Elijah McCoy, the Canadian inventor educated in Scotland, who invented an automatic lubricating cup which allowed trains to travel without the delays that were erstwhile necessary in order to add oil to the axles and bearings. Elijah's invention spawned many copies, all inferior to the original and so he patented the design in 1872.

Introduction

We do not have enough trained therapists to correctly diagnose and manage the tsunami of people who are being failed by 'conventional' medicine. Conventional medicine may provide the short-term relief of symptom-suppressing medication, and the short-term reassurance that 'something is being done', but it fails to address the underlying causes. The inevitable result is a progression of the underlying pathology, so that we have more chronically sick and dysfunctional adults and children than ever before.

I learned about the inadequacies of modern medicine through working with thousands of patients with chronic fatigue syndrome and myalgic encephalitis. Conventional medicine had and still has little to offer these pathologically fatigued patients. The correct treatment seems so obvious now, but when I first started talking about energy delivery mechanisms in the 1980s, I was considered unhinged. When this progressed to putting my ideas into the public arena in an online website,[†] I was attacked by mainstream doctors for such heretical ideas and subjected to endless investigation by the UK's General Medical Council (GMC). This was despite not a single complaint from a patient, not a single patient worsening as a result of my treatments, and not a single patient being put at risk of harm. A revealing comment arising from an FOIA (Freedom of Information) search came from the GMC's own barrister Mr Tom Kark: 'The problem with the Myhill cases is that all the patients are improved and none will give witness statements against her.'

The current 'football match' score is Myhill 38, GMC nil.[‡] In other words, there have been 38 GMC investigations concluded against me and all have found in my favour. My most recent GMC hearing was in Oct 2020, which I again won. Interested

---

[†]My website – www.drmyhill.co.uk – currently (as of September 2022) has had in excess of 24 million hits. I think it is a classic example of the Streisand Effect: this is a phenomenon that occurs when an attempt to hide, remove or censor information has the unintended consequence of increasing awareness of that information, often via the Internet. It is named after American singer, Barbra Streisand, whose attempt to suppress the California Coastal Records Project photograph of her residence in Malibu, California, taken to document California coastal erosion, inadvertently drew greater attention to it in 2003. So, by trying to put me out of action, the GMC drew attention to me, and people visited my site in their droves!

[‡]**Sporting aside:** The highest score in an English Football League match is 13-0 and that has been achieved three times. The first such occasion was on 6 January 1934 when Stockport County beat Halifax Town 13-0 in a Third Division (North) fixture. The Scottish Football Cup can do better – Arbroath beat Bon Accord 36–0 on 12 September 1885. But my 38-0 thrashing of the GMC outstrips them all; Craig has even had a polo shirt made up for me, with my GMC score emblazoned across the chest!

readers can learn more from my website.[1] At that point I relinquished my registration with the GMC because that gave me the clinical freedom to speak my mind without the bore of yet another investigation. What is so interesting is that I have continued to practise as a Naturopathic Physician but have been no less effective because I find the Tools of the Trade are available without doctors' prescription. They can all be found in Nature's pantry.

What to expect from this book

The thyroid gland is a vital part of energy delivery mechanisms. The underactive thyroid is now so common that it needs to be considered in the treatment of any chronic condition. Conventional medicine routinely misdiagnoses such cases and thereby delays diagnosis. Worse, when the diagnosis is made by physicians like myself, then conventional doctors obstruct, mislead and frighten patients into stopping their healing treatment.

- What this book is: It describes how we can all effectively and safely diagnose and treat our own underactive thyroid to reverse current pathology, improve quality of life and prevent future pathology.
- What this book is not: It is not a textbook. There will, however, be a fair smattering of supporting medical papers and references, all listed at the end of the book, by chapter. The reader can choose to look them up or just to plough on, safe in the knowledge that 'they are there'.

In essence this book is the path to living well and to your full potential. You have to do it yourself because your doctor will not do it for you.

Just do it!

Introducing the thyroid gland

Perhaps before we end this introduction, we should say a little about the thyroid gland itself. The word 'thyroid' is derived from the Latin 'thyreoidea' which can be traced back to the Ancient Greek word θυρεοειδής, meaning 'shield-like/shield-shaped'. The shape and location of the thyroid gland can be seen in Figure 1.

In the course of this book you will find out what it does, what may make it become

Figure 1.1: Position of thyroid in the neck

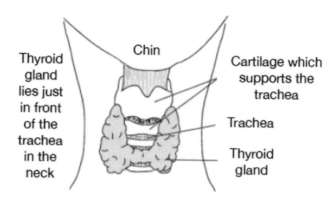

underactive and why that is important. Also how to spot for yourself if yours or a loved one's is under-performing, as most doctors today rely solely on blood tests and thereby miss many diagnoses, and how to support your thyroid back to health.

Part I

The practical

Chapter 1

Are you hypothyroid?
The symptoms and signs of an underactive thyroid

Listen to the patient, they will tell you the diagnosis

Sir William Osler

With respect to medical disorders, 90% of the diagnosis comes from the patient's history. Tests are helpful but, on their own, cannot be relied on. This is particularly true for managing the underactive thyroid and adjusting the dose of any replacement hormones. Understanding why symptoms arise is the starting point for proper diagnosis and management because we use symptoms to monitor the dose and timing. We need the full picture.*

The thyroid is a vital part of energy delivery mechanisms. I use the car analogy. For full function we need the right fuel in the tank (a paleo-ketogenic diet), the mitochondrial

---

*__Astronomical aside:__ One has to look very carefully to arrive at the full picture. As an analogy, consider Polaris, the North or Pole Star, so called because its current position is less than a degree away from the north celestial pole. The Ancients thought this to be the (single) brightest star in the constellation Ursa Minor, and as such it is designated *Alpha Ursae Minoris*. In fact, Polaris is a triple star system (three stars all orbiting each other), composed of the primary, a yellow supergiant designated *Polaris Aa*, in orbit with a smaller companion, *Polaris Ab* and then this pair is in a wider orbit with *Polaris B*. At one time there were thought to be two more widely separated components—*Polaris C* and *Polaris D* – but these have been shown not to be physically associated with the Polaris system. All this took time, effort, a lot of mathematics, many *different* methods of astronomical investigation, such as observation by the naked eye, observation through a variety of telescopes, the use of variable radial velocity calculations, and the determination of some very clever people – things had to be ruled in and things had to be ruled out. The same principles apply to diagnosing hypothyroidism – one has to look at lots of *different* factors, be determined and not rely on a single measure. Relying on such a single measure was the mistake the Ancients made with Polaris – their eyes saw one bright star and so they thought there was one bright star. Wrong! Conventional doctors see 'normal' blood test result(s) and so the patient does not 'have a thyroid problem'. (Often) wrong!

engine (see Chapter 3, a microcosm of our book *Diagnosis and Treatment of Chronic Fatigue Syndrome and Myalgic Encephalitis – it's mitochondria not hypochondria*) together with the control mechanisms of the thyroid accelerator pedal and the adrenal gearbox. The symptoms of the underactive thyroid are split into those that apply to poor energy delivery mechanisms and those that are specific to the thyroid. This distinction is important because to treat those general symptoms of poor energy delivery may well need attention to diet, gut function and mitochondrial and adrenal issues before one can effectively employ thyroid support.

Table 1.1: General symptoms of the underactive thyroid (which equally apply to poor diet and poor mitochondrial and adrenal function)

What	Symptoms and signs	Notes
Poor energy delivery to the body	Chronic fatigue syndrome/ myalgic encephalitis with poor stamina; all activities must be paced	Fatigue is pathological if energy is not restored after a good night's sleep
	The body runs cold	The enzymes of our mitochondrial engines need warmth to work well. We turn into sluggish poikilothermic[†] lounge lizards
	Intolerance of cold	Because the body is already running cold and colder translates to slower
	Intolerance of heat	We need extra energy to pump blood to the skin to lose heat, but this extra energy is not available when energy delivery mechanisms are down
	Obesity – for two reasons:	1. We do not burn so many calories, so these are stored as fat 2. Having no energy is very stressful. Many use addictions to help deal with stress. Addictions include the comfort eating of sugar, fruit sugar, carbs and junk food. Most people are carb addicts, and this results clinically in weight gain, high blood pressure and eventually diabetes. See our book *Prevent and Cure Diabetes*

Poor energy delivery to the brain	Foggy brain, poor short-term memory, inability to multitask or problem solve. In children this amounts to low IQ. Adults, often mental illness. Elderly, dementia	The brain weighs 2% of body weight but consumes 20% of all energy – it needs a lot of energy to work! Children so afflicted are called 'cretins'. Adults may progress to myxoedema madness (which starts with depression). Hypothyroidism is a major risk factor for dementia
	The brain gives us symptoms of slow energy expenditure, such as feeling stressed, depression, anxiety and procrastination	Stress is the symptom we experience when the brain knows it does not have the energy to deal with demands
Poor energy delivery leads to being 'unattractive'	We cherish people with lots of energy. They have fun and get things done. We learn to recognise the signs of that. This is part of 'beauty'‡	A happy person is a person with energy who bounces around and wants to do things. That is further reflected in an attractive, jolly, smiling face. We fall in love with energetic characters because energy has major evolutionary survival value
The use of addictions	The above symptoms are unpleasant. Addictions mask them	Obvious addictions include caffeine, alcohol, nicotine and other such. However, the most pernicious addiction is to sugar, fruit sugar and refined carbohydrates, i.e. 'junk food'. This is socially acceptable, cheap, convenient and confers instant (short-term) relief but it is not sustainable and leads to disease escalation
Poor energy delivery to the immune system which leads to:		

†**Footnote:** A 'poikilotherm' is an organism (such as a frog) with a variable body temperature that tends to fluctuate with, and is similar to or slightly higher than, the temperature of its environment.

‡The words 'attractive' and 'beauty' may seem unusual terms to find in a description of the symptoms and signs of illness, but I use these because they are universally 'understood', not in any 'judgemental' or 'discriminatory' way. The fact is that we 'look different' when we are ill, and evolution has 'taught' us to recognise these outward signs of illness as 'unattractive' – dark circles under the eyes, for example. Many of my most ill patients have become, as they have got better, the most attractive human beings.

Table 1.1 (cont'd)

What	Symptoms and signs	Notes
1. susceptibility to infections	If the immune system does not deal effectively with acute infections, these may become chronic and switch on myalgic encephalitis (ME)	The immune system needs large amounts of energy to deal with infection (see our book *The Infection Game*)
2. slow healing and repair	The gut lining, bone marrow, skin and hair are grown and replaced daily so we see:	We know this because these rapidly dividing cells are most impacted by cancer chemotherapy, which destroys energy-delivery mechanisms
	- poor quality hair, skin and nails	Insufficient energy for fast growth
	- gut problems – leaky gut (see below), allergies, inflammation	Insufficient energy for a healthy lining to the gut
	- anaemia (in an estimated 20-60% of hypothyroid patients)	Insufficient energy for making red blood cells. Often the red cells are larger than normal, but there are fewer of them
	- low numbers of white cells	This further contributes to poor immunity
	- platelets are larger and stickier	This increases the risk of thrombosis
	- accelerated ageing with organ failures (heart, brain, renal etc) and degeneration (arthritis, osteoporosis)	We inevitably damage our bodies by day, and healing and repair take place by night. If the rate of damage exceeds the rate of repair, we degenerate
Inflammation	Where there is leaky gut there is potential for gut bacteria, fungi and viruses to leak into the bloodstream and body tissues. This drives inflammatory reactions at distal sites	I suspect this is a driver of many arthritic conditions (including polymyalgia rheumatica), temporal arteritis, venous ulcers, inflammatory bowel disease, intrinsic asthma, kidney disease, myocarditis, irritable bladder and possibly psychosis. And, of course, cancer

Table 1.2: Symptoms more specific to the thyroid

Mechanism	Symptom	Notes
Fluid retention and oedema	Puffy face	Compare current looks with old photographs
	Large tongue	You may see indentations from where teeth lie against the tongue
	Obstructive sleep apnoea, perhaps with snoring	Because the tissues of the throat are swollen, and this constricts the airways
	Voice changes	The vocal cords are puffy
	Swollen, puffy legs, most obvious in the ankles at the end of the day	A cause of 'non-pitting oedema'
	Problems with 'trapped nerves' e.g. carpal tunnel syndrome, sciatica	Swollen tissues squash nerves
Poor fat burning	Ketogenic hypoglycaemia – on a PK diet you need thyroid hormones to burn fat; if low, then fat burning is done with adrenalin and this gives all the symptoms of low blood sugar	The symptoms of low blood sugar are not due to low blood sugar but to the adrenalin (and other hormonal) pumped out in response to low blood sugar
	Gaining weight despite being on a keto diet – this may point to hypothyroidism	You need thyroid hormones to burn fat
Sleep disturbance	Poor quality, unrefreshing sleep	This is well recognised in hypothyroidism but the mechanism is uncertain. It may be in part sleep disturbance due to ketogenic hypoglycaemia
	Being an owl (drop off to sleep late, wake late) and so feeling 'jet-lagged'	There are at least three groups of hormones for quality sleep and correct diurnal rhythm – melatonin, TSH and T4/T3. Light inhibits melatonin production, dark stimulates such. Melatonin stimulates the pituitary and so TSH spikes at midnight. Then T4 spikes at 4:00 am, T3 at 5:00 am, which stimulates the production of adrenal hormones that wake you up

Table 1.2 (cont'd)

Mechanism	Symptom	Notes
Proximal myopathy – that is, symmetrical weakness of 'proximal' (upper) and/or lower limbs	This may present with difficulty climbing hills or stairs, trouble getting out of the bath or off the floor or even up from a chair… or getting on to a horse! Press-ups become impossible	Often misdiagnosed as lack of fitness
Poor energy delivery plus oedema of the gut?	Constipation	Constipation is often an early symptom to improve once the underactive thyroid has been corrected. I am not sure of the mechanism of this but it is probably a combination of poor energy delivery, being cold and oedema of the gut
Uncertain	Headaches	Again, I am not sure of the mechanism of this but clinically, headaches often settle

Table 1.3: Signs of poor energy delivery mechanisms (the combined effects of poor diet and poor mitochondrial, thyroid and adrenal function) – useful for diagnosing and monitoring

Symptom	Mechanism	Notes
Low core temperature – that is, below 36.6°C (97.88°F)	Poor energy delivery	Monitoring core temperature is helpful to get the dose of thyroid and adrenal supplements right – see Chapter 4
Low blood pressure – that is, below 110/70 mm Hg	Poor energy delivery to the heart so it cannot beat powerfully	This may well be masked by the adrenalin of metabolic syndrome (a pre-diabetic condition) or ketogenic hypoglycaemia
Slow pulse – that is, less that 70 bpm in a non-athlete	The thyroid is largely responsible for the resting pulse rate	A normal person, not in athletic training, should have a resting pulse of 70-75 bpm. Again, this may be masked by adrenalin as above

Table 1.4: Medical history of the underactive thyroid – useful for suspecting the diagnosis

What	Why	Notes
Being female	Taking the Pill and HRT are major risk factors for the underactive thyroid	Women with CFS/ME outnumber men by at least 4:1 – see www.meresearch.org.uk/ sex-differences-in-mecfs and paper by Baha Arafah, 2001, which has the telling conclusion: 'In women with hypothyroidism treated with thyroxine, estrogen therapy may increase the need for thyroxine.'[1]
Family history	Thyroid problems run in families	Possibly genetic[2] but families have the same diet, environmental and infectious exposures. Genetic risk does not mean that there is nothing that can be done
Other autoim-mune conditions	Autoimmunity runs in families[2]	Again, possibly genetic but, again, families have the same diet, environmental and infectious exposures
Gradual decline into ill health	The thyroid may be slowly destroyed by autoimmunity, micronutrient deficiency, toxins, radiation...	All the above symptoms are ascribed by doctors to age, stress, menopause, etc so patients are dismissed without proper clinical consideration. This is further reason to do it yourself
	...and prescription medica-tions	Lithium,[3] amiodarone[4] and beta blockers[5] have been clearly linked but there are probably many others
Triggers:		Be aware of the increased risk if any of the following are in your medical history
1. vaccines	These are good at triggering autoimmune disease	See the list of 31 studies below that demon-strate that vaccines can trigger autoimmune responses. For a more recent report, specific to thyroid function, see Vera-Lastra et al's 2021 report[6]
2. menopause	Progesterone increases the efficacy of thyroid hormones	The menopause may unmask underlying hypothyroidism. In consequence many women have been wrongly prescribed progesterone (when the underactive thyroid diagnosis has been missed) and this is dangerous medicine as progesterone is carcinogenic

Table 1.4 (cont'd)

What	Why	Notes
3. viral infection	May present with an overactive thyroid and this progresses to an underactive thyroid, typically in women aged 40-50 triggered in summer and early autumn	So called sub-acute thyroiditis (SAT) – for example, there is evidence of SAT being preceded by upper respiratory tract infection, of elevated viral antibody levels, and of both seasonal and geographical clustering of cases[7]
4. whiplash injury	A good friend and osteopath has noticed this association	This is biologically plausible as there may well be soft tissue injury in the neck

Having established the clinical picture suggesting an underactive thyroid, then we can do laboratory tests to support that suggestion.

The evidence base for the relationship between immune responses and vaccinations

Here is a list of medical papers showing the link between allergic and autoimmune responses and vaccinations:

1. Shoenfeld & Aron-Maor 2000.[8]
2. Nossal, 2000.[9]
3. Shoenfeld, Aron-Maor and Sherer, 1996.[10]
4. Cohen & Shoenfeld, 1996.[11]
5. Rogerson & Nye, 1990.[12]
6. Haschulla et al, 1990.[13]
7. Biasi et al, 1993.[14]
8. Biasi et al, 1994.[15]
9. Gross et al, 1995.[16]
10. Cathebras et al, 1996.[17]
11. Maillefert et al, 1999.[18]
12. Grasland et al, 1998.[19]
13. Pope et al, 1998.[20]
14. Tudela, Marti & Bonanl, 1992.[21]

15. Finielz & Lam-Kam-Sang, 1998.[22]
16. Guiseriz, 1996.[23]
17. Mamoux & Dumont, 1994.[24]
18. Grezard, et al, 1996.[25]
19. Weibel & Bemor, 1996.[26]
20. Ray et al, 1997.[27]
21. Howson & Fineberg, 1992.[28]
22. Howson et al, 1992.[29]
23. Mitchell et al, 1998.[30]
24. Mitchell et al, 2000.[31]
25. Nussinovitch, Harel & Varsano, 1995.[32]
26. Thurairajan et al, 1997.[33]
27. Maillefert et al, 2000.[34]
28. Adachi, D`Alessio and Ericsson, 2000.[35]
29. Older et al, 1999.[36]
30. Kennedy, 1999.[37]
31. Hogenesch et al, 1999.[38]

Finally, it is biologically plausible that the Covid-19 vaccines will switch on auto-immunity.[39]

Chapter 2

Blood tests for the underactive thyroid

Blood tests for the underactive thyroid have become the only route by which doctors generally are prepared to diagnose and monitor hypothyroidism, just as naked eye observation was the only way the Ancients (incorrectly) determined the nature of Polaris. In consequence, the diagnosis is often missed or delayed. Just as bad, replacement therapy may be inadequate because simply relying on blood tests means that under-dosing is common. Late diagnosis and under-dosing consign the patient to years of misery together with the increased risk of major pathology (see Chapter 9). I suspect one reason is intellectual idleness: it is so much quicker and easier to diagnose a condition with a fleeting and unthinking look at a piece of paper rather than take a proper medical history, as detailed in Chapter 1 – less work for doctors, which means that patients can be shovelled through the system in two instead of 20 minutes. Jolly good for out-patient vital statistics.*

Big Pharma too loves patients to be under-dosed because this leads to more pathology, more prescriptions and more profits. This has 'worked' very well for Big Pharma – as of

*Historical aside: Everything in the British NHS seems driven by meeting targets. Whilst targets have their place, they have to be drawn up and thought through very carefully so as not to end up being yet another example of the Law of Unintended Consequences. For example, the Soviet Union employed the idea of 'Five Year Plans' in order to control its economy. One target, many echelons down from the macro-targets of growth and GDP, was what length of steel plate certain factories should produce each quarter. The targets were set too high and so the only way the factory workers could meet the length targets was to reduce the thickness of the steel plate. This meant that the steel plate was too weak for the structures it was intended for and so buildings and machinery which used this weakened steel fell down and cracked apart. The analogy is clear – outpatient targets are the length of steel targets, and making the steel thinner is equivalent, here, to assessing the patient quickly (not delving too deep; being 'thin' in your investigations) and ultimately, the steel fails, and causes problems further down the line, just as the patient risks major pathology in later life from poor diagnosis methods early on.

end-2020, the total global pharmaceutical market was valued at about US$1.27 trillion, having made striking increases from its 2001 valuation of US$390 billion.[1]

Doctors have been able to get away with this sloppy approach because the onset of the underactive thyroid is usually slow and insidious. The Soviet factory workers in the Historical aside also got away with it until the buildings fell down and the machinery cracked. It is all too easy to blame other factors for hypothyroid symptoms: you are stressed, menopausal, overweight, unfit, old… when of course these are often the very symptoms of the underactive thyroid! Dr Kenneth Blanchard, consultant endocrinologist, reckons that at least 20% of all Western women are hypothyroid.[2] There are many different quoted rates of prevalence but, for example, *Science Direct* reports that 'in the United States [the rate] among white women is 5.8%, and is 5.3% and 1.2% among Hispanic-American and African-American women, respectively'.[3] This means there must be many missed cases.

Even the blood tests can be misleading and misinterpreted, as shown in Table 2.1.

Table 2.1: Usual tests for thyroid function and their limitations

Blood test	What I consider to be a normal range	The problem	Notes
TSH (thyroid stimu-lating hormone)	Less than 1.5 mIU/l	Often this is the only test done but it only picks up a *primary* failure of the thyroid gland	Most of my patients with CFS/ME have *secondary* hypothyroidism due to poor pituitary function. With pituitary (or secondary) hypothyroidism, expect to see the TSH suppressed: e.g. <0.01 mIU/l. Hence it is essential to look at the free T4 and free T3 levels also
		The reference range for a normal result is set too high. In UK some doctors will not prescribe until the TSH is above 10 mIU/l	In the USA the threshold for prescribing is a TSH above 3.0 mIU/l. For pregnant women the threshold for prescribing is above 1.5 (see Chapter 7). I have never understood the logic for this – why the problem level in pregnant women should not also be a problem in other people. That is why I like to see TSH of <1.5 mIU/l

		The TSH level is often used to monitor the dose of thyroid hormones	For all the reasons above, this results in long-term under-dosing
T4 (thyroxine)		This is affected by protein binding so do not rely on T4 levels – always ask for a 'free T4' test	Oestrogen in the Pill and HRT increases thyroid binding globulin, and this may lower the free T4
Free T4 (FT4)	12-24 pmol/l	This wide population reference range is not the same as one's individual reference range	Someone whose personal reference range may be 20-22pmol/l would be told they were normal should the result be 12pmol/l We do not know what anyone's personal reference range is. We can only find out through a trial of thyroid replacement treatment, with clinical and biochemical monitoring. Professor Sir Antony Toft, in his book *The British Medical Association Guide to Treating Hypothyroidism*, states that some do not feel well until their FT4 is running at 30 pmol/l. Even population reference ranges only encompass 95% of individuals; some who are hypothyroid will still be judged as 'normal' if levels run above or below this range. Again, clinical input – the doctor talking with and examining the patient – is vital
			The 'half-life' of thyroxine is 9-10 days,[4] so the timing of a blood test is not critical, unlike T3 (see below)
T3 (triiod-othyro-nine)		Again, this is affected by protein binding so do not rely on T3 levels – always ask for a 'free T3' test	
Free T3 (FT3)	3.2-6.8 pmol/l	The population reference range is not the same as one's individual reference range	We do not know what anyone's personal reference range is. We can only find out through a trial of thyroid replacement treatment, with clinical and biochemical monitoring

Table 2.1 (cont'd)

Blood test	What I consider to be a normal range	The problem	Notes
		T3 is the active hormone	So, one could have a high freeT4, but if the free T3 were low you might still be underactive. This is called 'T3 hypothyroidism'
			The 'half–life' of T3 is much shorter (compared with T4) – probably about 24 hours.[5] According to *Science Direct* again, liothyronine reaches its maximum efficacy within the first 24 hours of administration and is thus the quickest of the the thyroid hormones to take effect. In normal circumstances, T3 has a half life of around two days. For comparison purposes, you should allow roughly the same time between dosing with T3 (or thyroid glandular) and the blood test – say six to 12 hours – each time you test. This also means thyroid glandular needs to be taken at least twice daily – on rising and at midday
Reverse T3 (rT3) – see below	0.13-0.35 nmol/l	If this inactive from of T3 is high, this points to thyroid hormone receptor resistance. In this event, the blood tests are not helpful. NHS labs rarely measure rT3 yet a high level nullifies all the above	Given the possibility of hormone receptor resistance, all the more reason to monitor using primarily clinical (symptoms and signs) rather than biochemical parameters

What is 'reverse T3'?

T4 is capable of being converted into either T3 (active thyroid hormone) or reverse T3 (metabolically inactive), depending on the removal of specific iodine atoms. Normally, roughly 40% of T4 is converted into T3 and about 20% into reverse T3. However, if the thyroid is malfunctioning, or if the body needs to conserve energy or is under significant stress, the conversion ratio may change to, say, 50% of T4 being converted to reverse T3. A significant change such as this greatly impacts thyroid function and hormone availability. It does this because reverse T3 and T3 compete for the same receptors throughout the body. If there is a greater prevalence of reverse T3 in the system, it will effectively block active thyroid hormone from reaching cells – that is, lead to high thyroid hormone receptor resistance. This means that, without reverse T3, there is a risk that T3 levels will become dangerously high, resulting in *hyper*thyroidism. Alternatively, too much reverse T3 overly inhibits active T3, and at the same time nullifies all other test results because hormone receptor resistance is high, thus skewing all other blood test readings – whatever the levels of TSH, T4 and T3, the cells cannot respond.

How to assess thyroid activity when blood tests are unreliable

For all the reasons described in Table 2.1, the patient may be in the invidious position of being told that their test results are normal, even when these lie only just within the population normal range, and/or even when their normal range does not coincide with the population normal range, and/or when they are suffering from numerous clinical symptoms and have many clinical signs to suggest otherwise.

Even so, thyroid function blood tests should be done in every case before using thyroid glandular (TG) for two reasons:
1.   To make sure you do not have an overactive thyroid.
2.   To see is there is biochemical scope for a trial of TG.

Where the problem is thyroid hormone receptor resistance, blood tests are worthless, and all the monitoring must be clinical. Thankfully this is uncommon and usually improves with detoxification regimes (see Chapter 6).

There are other blood tests that may support the diagnosis of the underactive thyroid and/or these should be done to screen for related issues. These are set out in Tables 2.2 and 2.3.

Autoimmunity and thyroid problems

Table 2.2: Blood tests for autoimmunity

What	Why	Notes
Auto-antibodies	Any positive result is always abnormal	Laboratories often give a 'normal' reference range as if it is regarded as acceptable to have some antibodies. This is not acceptable! Any autoantibodies are abnormal – they amount to the immune system being in a state of civil war and attacking self
Thyroglobulin antibody (TGA)	This knocks out thyroid globulin, which is essential for hormone synthesis	Both TGA and TPO (see next) can be abnormal in the underactive and the overactive thyroid
Thyroid peroxidase antibody (TPO)	This knocks out one of the enzymes that make thyroid hormones	TPO is present in: 60% of cases of Graves' disease 90% of cases of Hashimoto's thyroiditis (often at high levels) 80% of cases of primary myxoedema[6, 7, 8]
Antibodies to the TSH receptor	These result in uncontrolled stimulation of the thyroid leading to thyrotoxicosis	These antibodies are rarely measured but may be high with the overactive thyroid

The common risk factors for thyroid antibodies are iodine deficiency, vaccination, vitamin D deficiency, the Pill and HRT, Western diets especially consumption of gluten and dairy, and fluctuating blood sugar levels – see, for example, references 9, 10, 11 and 12 (page 208) plus the 31 studies concerning autoimmunity and vaccination in the previous chapter (page 10).

Having one autoimmune disease increases the risk of others. Cojocaru et al concluded in 2010 that: 'Disorders of autoimmune pathogenesis occur with increased frequency in patients with a history of another autoimmune disease'.[13]

With that understanding, correct these risk factors with Lugol's iodine (chapter 13), vitamin D 10,000 IU daily and the PK diet, and avoid vaccination.

Other factors

Table 2.3: Other blood test results which may suggest a diagnosis of hypothyroidism

What	Why	Notes
High total cholesterol – that is, above 7 mmol/l	Due to increasing levels of the 'unfriendly' LDL cholesterol	Cholesterol abnormalities are a symptom, not a cause, of arterial disease. When the thyroid goes slow, the immune system goes slow, so healing and repair of arteries goes slow. The liver pushes out more cholesterol to assist this healing and repair process
		High total cholesterol is also a symptom of vitamin D deficiency simply because vitamin D is synthesised in the skin through the action of sunshine on cholesterol. It is completely safe, and indeed desirable, for adults to take vitamin D 10,000 IU daily; children under 12 years can take 5000 IU and babies 1000 IU
Large red blood cells – that is, above 95 fl	Poor bone marrow function due to poor energy delivery	Also possibly due to poor assimilation of vitamins B12 and B9 (folic acid)

Table 2.3 (cont'd)

What	Why	Notes
High homocysteine – a normal level is below 10 mcmol/l		With large red blood cells, it is vital to measure homocysteine which is a major risk factor for arterial disease, cancer and dementia.[14, 15, 16] According to Wu and Lu (2002), plasma homocysteine is a risk factor for coronary heart disease, and also increases the chances of developing cancer.[15] Levels come down reliably well with B vitamins. Strain et al concluded in 2004 that the single largest (nutritional) reason for raised plasma homocysteine is folate (vitamin B9) deficiency. They also concluded that vitamin B12, and to a lesser extent vitamin B6, lowered plasma homocysteine[17]
		To correct a high homocysteine level, you need the following methylated B vitamins daily for life: pyridoxal 5 phosphate 50 mg (in most good multivitamins) methyl folic acid (MTHFA) 800 mcg methylated B12 3 mg glutathione 250 mg This usually does the trick but some people need methyl B12 by injection, so retest after four months of the above
Anaemia with low haemoglobin and low numbers of red blood cells	Poor bone marrow function due to poor energy delivery	Wherever there is anaemia, always think of blood losses from the gut due to pathology and measure faecal occult blood and faecal calprotectin
Low white blood cell count	Poor bone marrow function due to poor energy delivery	This may be masked if the immune system is trying to fight a chronic infection and trying to push out more white cells
Large platelets	Probably again poor bone marrow function due to poor energy delivery	Look for high mean platelet volume (MPV) and high platelet distribution width (PDW)

Low ferritin – that is, low iron	You need an acid stomach to absorb iron. Hypothyroidism leads to hypochlorhydria – that is, low stomach acid and therefore poor absorption of nutrients	With low stomach acid, there is malabsorption of iron, and indeed many other minerals

In conclusion

It is a combination of the clinical picture (symptoms and signs) and the biochemical tests (Tables 2.1, 2.2 and 2.3) that allow us to hypothesise hypothyroidism. However, the proof of the pudding lies in response to treatment with a trial of thyroid glandular (TG), yet before such a trial can start we must first put the body in a fit state to respond.... Read on!

But before you read on, dear reader, the authors acknowledge that this chapter is a bit 'heavy', even with the distraction of Soviet steelmakers, and so here is a little Romantic Interlude' with which we would like to conclude:

Romantic interlude

Those who regularly travel the London Underground will be used to the 'Mind the Gap' announcements made when the train doors are opening and closing. But how many have noticed that the voice is *very different* at Embankment Station, Northern Line? Here, and only here, you will hear Oswald Laurence, actor, deceased 2007, pronounce 'Mind the Gap' in his distinctive and very English voice. Why? Dr Margaret McCollum was wife to Oswald, and she used to frequently travel via Embankment and used to love hearing her husband's voice on the tannoy. But then Oswald died and London Underground changed all its announcements to a new digital system. No longer could Margaret listen to Oswald. After many requests by Margaret, and much to-ing and fro-ing and searching of their recording archives, London Underground 'found' Oswald and restored him to Embankment, Northern Line. Nowadays, Margaret goes down the tube not on her way to work, because she is now retired, but instead, just to listen to her husband's voice. (See 'Secret London' for more detail[18] and hear Oswald on youtube.[19])

Chapter 3

Before you start a trial of thyroid glandular (TG)

Taking thyroid hormones works because they kick the body, brain and immune system into action. This means we have to first put these organs into a fit state to respond; otherwise, we are flogging a dead horse.

Remember, and I repeat, the thyroid is a vital part of energy delivery mechanisms. I use the car analogy. For full function we need the right fuel in the tank (a paleo-ketogenic diet), and the mitochondrial* engine (see below), together with the control mechanisms of the thyroid accelerator pedal and the adrenal gearbox:

- First, we have to put the right fuel in the tank: diet and gut function.
- Second, we have to tune the mitochondrial engine.
- *Then* we balance up the thyroid accelerator pedal and the adrenal gearbox.

In that order.†

*__Explanatory note__: Mitochondria are often referred to as the powerhouses of the cell. They help turn the energy we take from food into energy that the cell can use. All multi-cellular eukaryotic organisms (organisms whose cells contain a nucleus and other membrane-bound organelles), from peanuts and pineapples to porcupines and professors, have mitochondria, and central to the function of mitochondria is this conversion of food into energy that can be used by the organism. For the biologists, prokaryotes (organisms whose cells lack a nucleus and other organelles) – bacteria and 'archaea' – do not have mitochondria, but all eukaryotes do.

†__Historical aside:__ Roman scholars and engineers often used phrases to emphasise the need to do things in the correct order so as to get the correct results – for example, road building needed certain layers of different substances to be laid down in a certain order to achieve a road that would (ultimately) last centuries. One such phrase was: *a solis ortu usque ad occasum* (from sunrise to sunset) meaning that days followed a set order and so should we. This saying was later interpreted as the monarch's dominion over lands, and by the Spanish Empire, and later the British Empire, as being 'empire[s] on which the sun never sets', the latter still being technically accurate as of 2021.[1]

1. The right fuel in the tank

First, we have to put the right fuel in the tank. This means attending to our diet and gut function.

The human gut has evolved and adapted to deal with a paleo-ketogenic (PK) diet – that is, a diet that follows 'paleo' principles and uses 'ketones' for fuel, as I will explain. It is high in unprocessed fat and plant fibre.

Such a diet supplies our mitochondrial engines with the perfect fuel of ketones which come either from fat or from the fermentation of fibre by friendly microbes in the large bowel. Our mitochondria – the micro-structures in nearly all our cells that produce energy – can use both fats and sugars as fuel. They can deal with sugars and carbohydrates for the short autumnal window of time when we have windfalls of fruit, nuts, vegetables and seeds. Indeed, in the very short term, sugars are rocket-fuel. However, relentless rocket-fuel burns out our engines and damages our bodies, resulting in accelerated ageing and premature disease. It is vital for health that we spend most of our lives in ketosis.

I have devoted whole books to the paleo-ketogenic diet. You can get started with Appendix C (page 121). For further details of how many calories, how much protein, fat, fibre and much more nitty gritty, you need our book *Paleo-Ketogenic – the why and the how*. The PK diet is the single most important intervention, but also the most difficult. The main reason for difficulty is carbohydrate addiction and again you can read more in our book *Prevent and Cure Diabetes*. Type 2 diabetes can be cured, type 1 greatly improved, and type 3 (dementia) rendered reversible by adopting a PK diet.

If you are *not* prepared to go PK, then please stop reading now and pass this book onto someone who is. Yes! I am an old woman, irritable, grumpy[‡] and not prepared to waste time on the bleedin' obvious.

Keto flu and ketogenic hypoglycaemia

Once your diet is sufficiently low-carb, it may take a week to get into ketosis. This is because the body will always burn up those nasty dangerous sugars before utilising

---

[‡]**Note from Craig:** I have almost, but not quite, given up, on interjecting at such points, by reminding all and sundry, that Sarah is not old, not irritable, and not grumpy, but she does, however, hate to waste time. So, I shall leave it there, as to say more would be a waste of time!

those safe ketones. Normally the body switches into fat burning using thyroid hormones. However, if there is insufficient thyroid hormone, or the body has yet to 'learn fat burning', it will use adrenalin instead. In the short term this is called 'keto flu' (body yet to learn) but if it persists then this is ketogenic hypoglycaemia (body has insufficient thyroid). This gives you a powerful clue that you are hypothyroid.

The point here is that the symptoms of low blood sugar are not caused just by low blood sugar; many result from the adrenalin needed to switch on fat burning to supply fuel. The symptoms of low blood sugar are poor energy delivery symptoms (fatigue, foggy brain, etc – see Chapter 2) and 'wired but tired' adrenalin symptoms – inability to relax, disturbed sleep, feeling shaky, possibly fast heart rate with palpitations, and more.

If keto flu persists for more than two weeks, then it is likely you have ketogenic hypoglycaemia. Start taking thyroid glandular straight away, as detailed in Chapter 5. But do not skip the rest of this chapter and do read the next chapter too. It all has to be done!‡

The fermenting upper gut

Next, take vitamin C to bowel tolerance to deal with the fermenting upper gut (and incidentally much more). All who consult me, bar a rare and select few, are carbohydrate addicts, primarily fuelling their bodies with sugars and starches.¶ Fruit is a bag of sugar; whole grains, pulses and root vegetables are digested to sugar in the gut. Eventually, the ability of the gut to cope is overwhelmed and we develop a fermenting gut. This is the start of the slippery slope to ill-health and disease. Why?

---

§**Historical note:** This is like the Roman engineer finding a clay-ridden stretch of land where they are building a road and therefore needing to lay down more stones than usual, but still carrying on with the order of the remaining layers thereafter.

¶**Note from Craig:** Before becoming 'PK-adapted', crisps were my addiction. I ate at least six normal-sized bags of ready-salted crisps each and every day. (See how, even now, I try to rationalise this addiction by using the phrase 'normal-sized' as though I am saying to my inner self, 'It wasn't that bad'!) I even had a stash of 12 bags in my wardrobe, 'just in case'. I gave up crisps overnight. One Monday, I threw away all 'my' crisps, stashed in various rooms of our house, and I have not eaten even a single crisp since then. I know that eating even one packet will trigger the addiction and so I simply never eat them.
PS: Whenever I start something new, I always start on a Monday. I never start on a Tuesday, following my mother's frequently expressed advice of: 'Nothing new on a Tuesday', although I now realise that this was aimed at (not) wearing new clothes. See 'Why you shouldn't wear new clothes on a Tuesday'²

The human gut is almost unique in the mammal world. The upper gut is a sterile carnivorous gut (like a dog's), designed for digesting protein and fat. The lower gut is a fermenting vegetarian gut designed to utilise fibre (like a horse's except humans cannot ferment fibre that has very tough cellulose, such as grass). This allows humans to deal with many different foods and partly explains our success as a species. This system works perfectly until we overwhelm our ability to deal with sugars and starches by consuming too much. When this overwhelming happens, bacteria and yeasts colonise the hitherto sterile upper gut and start fermenting. This creates nasty symptoms and pathology. How come?

1. Foods are fermented to toxins such as ethyl, propyl and butyl alcohols, D lactate, ammonia compounds, hydrogen, hydrogen sulphide and much else. This fermentation is otherwise known as the 'auto-brewery syndrome'. All these nasties have the potential to poison us, and this includes giving us a 'foggy brain'. I just need a glass of wine to appreciate that fact!

2. Colonies of bacteria and fungi build up and are then further colonised by viruses (so called bacteriophages). Fermenting microbes produce bacterial endotoxins, fungal mycotoxins and viral particles. These toxins spill over into the portal vein, the blood vessel that connects our gut to the liver. The liver uses up much energy and raw materials to deal with these toxins. This is debilitating.

3. The gases generated by upper gut fermentation cause burping and bloating. They may distend the gut, and this is painful.

4. Microbes move into the lining of the gut and this low-grade inflammation results in leaky gut. This means that acid cannot be concentrated in the stomach because it leaks out as fast as it is secreted in. (The acid – hydrogen ions – are pumped into the lumen of the stomach from the bloodstream, by proton pumps in the stomach lining. This leaves behind an alkaline blood. When the protons leak back, the bloodstream returns to normal pH.) Acid is an essential part of digestion because:

    i)   it is essential to start the digestion of protein.

    ii)   it is necessary to absorb minerals.

    iii)   it sterilises the upper gut and protects us from infections.

    iv)   it determines gut emptying. A non-acid stomach does not empty correctly and this drives reflux, oesophagitis, heartburn and hiatus hernia.

5. Microbes, dead and alive, and undigested foods leak into the bloodstream and drive disease at distal sites. This is a major cause of pathology from inflammatory bowel disease, arthritis , fibromyalgia, connective tissue disease, autoimmunity, interstitial cystitis, urticaria, venous ulcers, intrinsic asthma, kidney disease, and possibly psychosis and other brain pathologies, such as Parkinson's disease.
6. Chronic inflammation of the lining of the gut results in cancer, especially of the stomach and oesophagus. Both are on the increase. Diet is the main reason, followed by acid-blocking drugs. These drugs also drive osteoporosis.

Fermentation of fibre by friendly microbes should take place in the colon, the lower gut. The gases which result and make you fart are hydrogen and methane. These farts are odourless. Put a match to them and they will explode …not that I recommend this for diagnostic purposes! If your farts are offensive, then that is because you have overwhelmed your digestion upstream and proteins are being fermented in your colon – rotting meat stinks. Short gut transit time will have a similar effect. Professor Gibson, a food microbiologist from the University of Reading, divides people into 'inflammables' and 'smellies'[#] – the inflammables (hydrogen and methane) have normal gut fermentation and the smellies (hydrogen sulphide) do not.[3]

Treating the upper fermenting gut
In order of importance:
*   First starve the little wretches (the microbes, that is) out with a PK diet.
*   Then kill 'em with vitamin C to bowel tolerance (also see Appendix E). Ascorbic acid is the best and the cheapest form of vitamin C. I suggest using the powder form and adding this to your daily bottle of water so it is consumed little and often through the day. Start with 2 grams (g) and build up by 1 g a day until you start to get gut symptoms. The idea is that vitamin C arrives in the upper gut and contact-kills all fermenters there. The body absorbs what it needs for other functions – good antioxidant status, detoxing, dealing with systemic infection, killing cancer cells and

[#]**Note from Craig:** At my secondary school, Aylesbury Grammar School, the prevailing odour indicated that most boys were smellies. However, one boy, in Craig's class, was capable of, and regularly demonstrated at house parties, and in the sports changing rooms, his ability to light his own farts. We all considered this a gift from the Gods, a super-power! It is only now that I have put two and two together and realised that this boy went home for lunch where baked beans were his staple - lots of fibre which he fermented to the flammable methane and hydrogen in the lower gut.

more. Any vitamin C surplus to requirements remains in the gut and passes into the large bowel. Here, it will start to kill some of the friendly fermenters, which are then fermented by other friendlies to produce gurgling and offensive farts. Increasing the dose further causes diarrhoea. Gurgling and farts will do nicely to indicate you have arrived at bowel tolerance – you have arrived! Then reduce the dose to just below that unsociable dose at which gurgling and farts are produced. This is bowel tolerance and is usually about 8-10 g daily. The dose may change with age and circumstance – with an acute infection it can increase to 100 g or more, depending on the infection (see our book, *The Infection Game*). The rules are the same: take to bowel tolerance.

- Kill 'em with iodine. This similarly wonderful and safe multitasking tool also contact-kills all microbes. It must be taken away from vitamin C as iodine is an oxidising agent (electron acceptor) while vitamin C is a reducing agent (electron donor) – if taken together they 'knock each other out'. I therefore suggest increasing slowly to a single dose of 50 mg at night (see Chapter 13).
- Stimulate normal digestion by chewing mastic gum 350 mg after meals.

Now that you have a non-fermenting gut, you will be able to absorb nutritional supplements.

Nutritional supplements

I no longer bother with nutritional tests in those people not taking supplements because I know what the result will show – a wide range of deficiencies. There are many possible reasons for this, not limited to but including:
- Since the advent of intensive farming, soils have become increasingly depleted, with minerals passing into plants, animals and humans, and into the sewers with no recycling. Mineral-deficient plants cannot synthesise vitamins.
- Carbohydrate-based diets are toxic because of fermentation. Vitamins and minerals are gobbled up by fermenting microbes living within the gut.
- We are poisoned by chemicals added to food and water, and in the air. These are 'anti-nutrients'.

We should all take a good multivitamin and a multimineral, vitamin D (10,000 IU), vitamin C (at least 5 g, ideally to bowel tolerance) together with essential omega-6 and -3 fatty acids. Hemp oil has the perfect ratio of 4:1. Consume a dessertspoonful daily.

Finally, iodine deficiency is extremely common and a cause of primary hypothyroidism. Recommended daily amounts are set far too low. Iodine has many functions over and above thyroid needs (see Chapter 13). We should all take Lugol's iodine 15% 3 drops (approximately 50 mg) daily.

2. Addressing the mitochondrial engine

Now it is time to address the mitochondrial engine.

'Mitochondrion'* is the singular form of 'mitochondria', and derives from Greek roots *mitos*, 'thread', and *khondrion*, 'tiny granule'. And so, its name describes its appearance pretty much exactly.*

Who is likely to have poor mitochondrial function?

- Any person with pathological fatigue. Pathological fatigue is the hallmark of CFS/ME. It is characterised by delayed fatigue whereby if you overdo things, energy levels are not restored by a good night's sleep.
- Most people over the age of 70 as with age our biochemistry slows.
- Anybody with any pathology, from diabetes and dementia to cancer and coronaries.

Indeed, at the start of my medical career in the 1980s, mitochondria as pathological players were unheard of. Now I do not know of a pathology where mitochondria are not involved. As described, mitochondria are the energy suppliers of the body and without enough energy, all things can, and will, 'go wrong' at some time. As a quick reminder, the PK diet and then the mitochondria supply the energy, and then the adrenals and thyroid match energy delivery to energy demand on a day-by-day, hour-by-hour and minute-by-minute basis.

*Linguisic note: There are many words that accurately describe themselves – for example, the word 'word' is perhaps the most classic example - well it is a word! We also have 'polysyllabic' – well it is, isn't it?! And 'sesquipedalian', meaning long word, and deriving from the Latin, meaning 'a foot and a half'. Our wonderful publisher, Georgina Bentliff, will love the correctness of this example – 'unhyphenated' – well again, it is, isn't it (and always should remain so)?! But my favourite can best be described by this short conversation:

What's the word to describe a one-word sentence?

Monepic.

Oh yes, that's right. Thanks!

Back to mitochondria....

Fixing your mitochondria

Fix your mitochondria by:

- Putting the right fuel in the tank – you have done that with the PK diet.
- Sorting the fermenting gut with vitamin C and iodine. You have done that too. From an evolutionary perspective, mitochondria are derived from bacteria, and they have similar needs. The very supplements that feed mitochondria also feed bacteria.
- Taking the mitochondrial package of supplements. The bare minimum, in order of importance, is:
  - magnesium 300 mg (and vitamin D 10,000 IU for its absorption)
  - co-enzyme Q 10 100 mg
  - niacinamide (vitamin B3) 1500 mg
  - acetyl L carnitine 1 g

  PLUS

  - D-ribose 5-15 g as a rescue remedy if you really overdo things. BUT this must be part of your carb count in the PK diet and 1 g D-ribose equals 1 g of carbs.
- Get rid of mitochondrial inhibitors. The common ones include products of the upper fermenting gut. Statins, one of my most hated drugs, cause fatigue because they inhibit the body's production of co-enzyme Q 10. Mitochondria may be inhibited by prescription medications, social addictions, pesticides, toxic metals, volatile organic compounds and microbial products. It is beyond the scope of this book to go into all such and how to get rid of them – you may need to see our comprehensive book *Ecological Medicine* among other sources.[4]

Mitochondria will start to heal and repair as soon as you start taking the supplements. I reckon it takes four months to see the full benefit. So long as you do not have ketogenic hypoglycaemia, I suggest allowing at least one month of PK diet, vitamin C to bowel tolerance, Lugol's iodine up to 50 mg, the basic package (see Groundhog Basic, page 147) and the mitochondrial package of supplements. During this time, you may well see improvements in energy delivery symptoms and signs. Whilst improving, change nothing, carry on. However, if you get stuck at a point where your level of fatigue is still pathological then move on to a trial of thyroid glandular. Next chapter please!

A summary of what to do

Table 3.1: What to do, the order of such and why

Order	What	Why	Reference
1	MUST start with the PK diet Ensure you are in ketosis using a ketone breath meter	If you are eating starchy carbohydrates and sugars. you will have a fermenting gut. Taking supplements will feed a fermenting gut	Appendix C See also our book *Paleo-ketogenic: The why and the how*
2	Then take vitamin C, at least 5 g daily, probably more, little and often through the day up to bowel tolerance. And Lugol's iodine 15% 3 drops at night	This helps kill upper gut fermenters, facilitates the absorption of minerals, protects you from infection, helps detox and improves antioxidant status	Appendix E
3	Then take the Basic Package of supplements	Now you will absorb these well	Appendix D
4	Then take the mitochondrial package of supplements	Now you will absorb these well	This chapter
5	Put in place detox regimes	If you suspect a toxicity problem	Appendix F
6	Then balance up the adrenal gear box and thyroid accelerator pedals	These glands work by kicking mitochondria into action. You need mitochondria in a fit state to respond	Chapters 4 and 5
7	Consider tests to identify any possible infections	If you suspect an immunological hole in the energy bucket	See our book *The Infection Game: Life is an arms race*

Table 3.1 (cont'd)

Order	What	Why	Reference
8	Put in place physiological and psychological interventions to deal with any mind-body issues	If you suspect an emotional hole in the energy bucket	See our book *Diagnosis and Treatment of CFS and ME – it's mitochondria, not hypochondria*
Through-out			
	You must pace so you do not suffer post-exertional malaise	Chronic production of lactic acid inhibits mitochondria and slows recovery	See Millan et al, 2022[5]
	Expect a bumpy ride and to get worse initially	All the above may cause short-term worsening because of diet, detox and die-off reactions	Appendix G
	Be satisfied with gentle progress in the right direction	It takes six months for the body to heal and repair and this demands energy too	
	If you get stuck, join a workshop	See my Workshops for Ecological Medicine and Sales Website Workshops Page and Workshops Facebook Group	See * https://drmyhill.co.uk/ wiki/ Workshops_for_ Ecological_Medicine * www.salesatdrmyhill. co.uk/ workshops-41-c.asp * www.facebook.com/ groups /538787526898346

Chapter 4

The adrenal gearbox:
Symptoms, diagnosis and management of adrenal fatigue

> *To understand the nature of disease is the fundamental object of medicine, for knowledge about a thing is the best way to acquire power over it.*
> *The Stress of Life*, 1956, Hans Selye (1907 – 1982)

Life does not afflict us with easily won, predictable demands. Life comes with unexpected nasty little events like war, starvation, natural disasters, bereavement, pandemics, family pressures, bullying and much more. It may seem that some suffer more than others, that these hardships are not fairly spread, that the Fates* are fickle, but we will all meet with some misfortune.

> *There is not a man alive who has wholly escaped misfortune.*
> *Ουδείς δε θνητών ταις τύχαις ακήρατος.*
> *Heracles*, Euripides, 480 – 406 BC, Ancient Greek tragedian

*Classical note: The Fates are a common motif in many European polytheistic cultures, exemplifying that Man has always suffered, and that he has always tried to explain this suffering. Examples of such include Ancient Greek, Roman, Slavic, Norse and Baltic mythologies. The Fates determine the destiny of all humans, and metaphors, such as spinning fibres or weaving threads, are often used to express these determinations. The Fates are almost exclusively female and reappear in later literature – for example, the three witches in Macbeth are undoubtedly a reference to this motif. The Roman Fates were:
- Nona, who spun the thread of life from her distaff onto her spindle
- Decima, who measured the thread of life with her rod
- Morta, who cut the thread of life and chose the manner of a person's death.

Whilst we cannot escape all misfortunes, we can do our best to prepare for them, and to be in our best shape to be able to deal with them, and much of this preparation comes down to having the energy to be able to cope with all these stresses. Energy is our main weapon against what the Fates spin for us.

We need energy:

- to rise to the occasion and fight,
- to hunt or grow food,
- to find shelter,
- for security and warmth and
- to find friends and family.

In our modern lives, much of this boils down to having the energy to work and earn money. Failure to deal with these stresses properly results in disability, disease and death.

Professor Hans Selye was the first to address the physiological and pathological basis of stress together with the body's reaction to such. He described the pathological picture that resulted, which he called the 'general adaptation syndrome'. In the short term, he saw adrenal swelling as the adrenals upgraded production of, and poured out, their hormones; in the long term, with unremitting stress, he saw shrunken adrenal glands and shrunken immune systems with severe weight loss, culminating in death.

The pathological picture described by Selye was the same regardless of the stressor: overwhelming infection, sleep deprivation, cold exposure, chronic pain, emotional stress, starvation, social isolation, financial hardship, and much more. It really was a 'general syndrome'.

Professor Selye described what he saw, but not the 'how' the – mechanism that lay behind it. He compared the human experience with a car motoring along and finally wearing out: adrenal glands swelling in response to acute stress, healing and repairing with rest, but shrinking to a state of atrophy with 'burn out' following chronic, unremitting stress. I think we can explain that 'how' in terms of energy delivery mechanisms.

The importance of matching energy demands to energy delivery

From an evolutionary perspective, food was the main rate-limiting step. Starvation would result in poor energy delivery, disability, disease and death. Primitive woman spent most, perhaps all, of her time seeking and storing food. Only when food security was assured dared she build her home and family. Energy (and so food) was spent with great economy, just like the original Scrooge. Not a farthing was wasted. So, for example, as soon as dark descended, primitive woman could not work productively and so hibernated to save energy.

> *Darkness is cheap, and Scrooge liked it.*
> *A Christmas Carol*, Charles Dickens (1812 – 1870), English writer and social critic

Our primitive woman would have needed energy to hunt and harvest. To do this successfully, her mitochondrial engines needed to go faster. She used her thyroid accelerator pedal and her adrenal gearbox to supply just enough energy – too much and energy was wasted, too little and her goal was not achieved. The thyroid accelerator pedal 'base loaded', running faster during the day and the light summers, but slower through the night and the dark winters. The adrenal gearbox fired up the mitochondrial engines second by second with adrenalin, minute by minute with cortisol and hour by hour with DHEA (see page 37) and sex hormones, so our primitive woman could move seamlessly from first gear into overdrive, according to need, wasting nothing. The more efficiently she could do this, the less energy she wasted and the better her chances of survival and the chances of survival of her offspring. This would be a powerful driving evolutionary force for survival. No wonder the body evolved a perfect energy control system.

Stress and increased energy demands

Stress is invariably accompanied by a demand for more energy.

When energy is available, we can deal with whatever life chooses to throw at us. With energy we can do it all and surmount all demands and obstacles. This brings reward, satisfaction and survival. After such achievement we rest and recover.

If energy is not available in the short term, we cannot spend it because, if energy spending exceeds energy delivery, we die. There is no energy to power the heart and other organs. Indeed, this is how our first marathon runner died.[†]

To prevent us all from dying like our heroic Greek through an energy overspend, the body gives us nasty symptoms. These symptoms have to be very unpleasant – if not we could ignore them and go on spending energy. If you are not sure what these nasty symptoms are, re-read Chapter 1.

How to diagnose poor adrenal function (adrenal fatigue)

Mainstream medical doctors never diagnose adrenal fatigue. They only recognise complete adrenal failure – Addison's disease[‡] – and diagnose this on very low serum cortisol and a short synacthen test – that is, the degree to which serum cortisol rises in response to kicking the adrenals with adrenocorticotropic hormone (ACTH). However, complete adrenal failure is rare whereas reduced function is common. Again, you will need to sort yourself out.

Again, diagnosis is hypothesised on symptoms, signs and tests and confirmed by response to treatment.

[†]**Classical note:** After the Athenian victory at the Battle of Marathon, Athens reached great and prosperous new heights. Democracy blossomed and became the foundation of Western civilization. L Siegfried, a German philosopher, put it this way: 'When Greeks were fighting at Marathon against the spiritually unconnected mass of Persians, they were fighting as people who had clear awareness of the right for a free political life. The consciousness of mankind… was born at Marathon. We, the people of the West, must always kneel respectfully to the place where human dignity was established.' After the battle, legend has it that the Greek messenger, Philippides, ran from the battlefield at Marathon to Athens in order to relay the great news of victory. He had sufficient energy to say, 'We were victorious!' but then collapsed and died. He had overspent his energy reserves.

[‡]**Medical historical note:** Addison's disease is named after Thomas Addison (1793 – 1860), an English physician of Guy's Hospital, London. He also described Addisonian anaemia [aka 'pernicious anaemia'] (later confirmed as a blood disorder caused by a lack of vitamin B12) and further, he wrote extensively on the actions of poisons. He suffered from marked episodes of depression throughout his life and eventually committed suicide by suddenly throwing himself over a sea wall, whilst out walking with those attending to him. The *Brighton Herald* reported that his melancholy was 'resulting from overwork of the brain', and it does seem that Addison did not look after himself and that he did not match his own personal energy delivery with his own very considerable personal energy demands. A lesson to us all.

Mechanisms by which symptoms are produced

- **Poor energy-delivery symptoms:** Because the adrenals are an essential part of energy delivery mechanisms, adrenal fatigue may present with all the symptoms of poor energy delivery (again, see Chapter 1). A useful clinical measure of the sum total of energy-delivery mechanisms is core temperature. This makes perfect sense. Starvation, mitochondrial failure, the underactive thyroid and the underactive adrenals will all present with low core temperature, and for such to normalise, all aspects of energy delivery need to be addressed. By the time you are reading this, I shall assume that the PK diet is established, and that the mitochondria have been improved and are nearing normal. That leaves us with the thyroid accelerator pedal and the adrenal gear box, ergo the inability to rise to the occasion and deal with stress.
- **Being a night owl:** It is the combination of adrenalin and cortisol that wakes you up. This means that the person who has late surges of adrenalin and cortisol will only come to life during the late afternoon or maybe the evening.
- **Wired but tired:** As adrenal glands fatigue, those hormone levels that we measure clinically drop in a particular order – first sex hormones, then DHEA, followed by cortisol and finally adrenalin. Normally, the stimulating effects of adrenalin are mitigated by cortisol and DHEA. This does not happen with adrenal fatigue, which is I suspect the mechanism behind this symptom, with inability to drop off to sleep, poor quality sleep and exaggerated startle reflex.
- **Salt and water imbalance problems:** Adrenal fatigue can be associated with a craving for salt, tendency to dehydration, possibly frequency of micturition (needing to pee often), tendency to low blood pressure and muscle cramps. Regulation of salt and water balance occurs via steroid hormones, known as mineralocorticoids.
- **Inflammation:** Adrenal hormones control inflammation in the body. With adrenal fatigue there is a tendency to inflammatory conditions such as allergy and autoimmunity together with an increased susceptibility to infection.

Adrenal stress test (saliva)

This test measures levels of cortisol, DHEA (and melatonin on request) over 24 hours. This is the most useful test for adrenal function because salivary levels of DHEA and cortisol are accurate (arguably better than blood tests because they – blood tests – are skewed by protein binding and the stress of undergoing blood testing), tests can be done in the (usually) less stressful environment at home and they are easily available to all. Normally one expects to see high levels of cortisol and DHEA in the morning which fall as the day progresses. The level of DHEA should be commensurate with the cortisol. Patterns of abnormality are as listed in Table 4.1.

With regard to HRT and as referenced in Table 4.1, the 2019 open-access paper that appeared in the *Lancet* by the Collaborative Group on Hormonal Factors in Breast Cancer, concluded that:

The clinical relevance of the main findings lies in the magnitude of the absolute risks during and after MHT [menopausal hormone therapy] use for women who start MHT at ages 40–59 years, but the public health relevance depends additionally on the numbers of women previously and currently exposed. Although use of either type of MHT for less than 1 year was associated with little subsequent risk, for women of average weight in developed countries, 5 years of use, starting at age 50 years, would cause an appreciable increase in the probability of developing breast cancer at ages 50–69 years. About half the excess would be during the first 5 years of current use of MHT, and half would be during the next 15 years of past use. The absolute increase would be about 2·0 per 100 women (one in every 50 users) for oestrogen-plus-daily-progestagen MHT, 1·4 per 100 women (one in 70 users) for oestrogen-plus-intermittent-progestagen MHT, and 0·5 per 100 women (one in 200 users) for oestrogen-only MHT. There is little difference in the absolute excess incidence by age 70 associated with starting 5 years of MHT use at ages 45 years, 50 years, or 55 years. Thus, addition of a daily progestagen increases the excess risk of breast cancer from one in 200 users to one in 50 users.

And

The corresponding risks with 10 years of use starting at age 50 years would be about twice as great. In western countries there have been about 20 million breast cancers diagnosed since 1990, of which about 1 million would have been caused by MHT use.

Table 4.1: Interpretation of an adrenal stress test

Significant result	What it means	Action
Cortisol and/or DHEA spikes above the upper limit at any time of day	Indicates a stress response as DHEA 'follows' cortisol which 'follows' adrenalin	Identify the cause of the stress. The commonest cause is the falling blood sugar of metabolic syndrome in the patient who is not keto-adapted – i.e. do the PK diet *now*!
	The adrenal gland is working okay but it, and the whole body, is stressed. This is not sustainable in the long term, and a crash is on the horizon	Again, identify the cause of the stress. Look for ways to reduce the demands on your life – physical, mental, emotional, financial, social, infectious and so on
Low DHEA, normal cortisol	The adrenal gland is starting to fatigue	Ditto above. Start adrenal support as below
Very low DHEA, low cortisol	The adrenal gland is now very fatigued	Ditto above
- and 'wired but tired'	Adrenalin is the last hormone to go down; high levels are no longer mitigated by cortisol and DHEA	
- and poor quality sleep	Ditto above	Ditto above Consider melatonin 3-9 mg at night
- and flattening of the circadian rhythm	Points to hypothyroidism	Sort the thyroid (see Chapter 5)
All the above	Accompanied by falling levels of sex hormones with loss of libido. This is Nature telling you that you do not have the reserves and energy for procreation	Do not suppress symptoms with HRT – this is dangerous medicine. HRT is growth promoting (risk of cancer)[1], immunosuppressive (risk of infection) and pro-thrombotic (risk of heart attack and stroke)

Treatment of adrenal fatigue

There are two key steps to treatment. First take the pressure off the adrenals and feed them. Then reduce their workload with herbals and adrenal glandulars.

1. Take the pressure off the adrenals and feed them

Essentially, the adrenals get fatigued because the body does not have the energy to deal with demands. In the short term, much can be achieved on adrenalin, but this is not sustainable in the long term. Look for ways to reduce the demands on your life – nutritional, physical, mental, emotional, financial, social etc. The largest stress comes from addictions: carbohydrates, caffeine, alcohol, nicotine, etc.

The adrenal glands are restored with rest: good sleep, naps in the day, meditation, weekends and holidays. Make sure you give them this opportunity if you can.

The adrenals are also particularly demanding of vitamin B5, vitamin C, salt and fats. These are all part of the Groundhog Basic regime (see Appendix D). Cholesterol is the starting point to synthesise all glucocorticoids, mineralocorticoids and sex hormones, as shown in Figure 4.1.

2. Reduce the work of the adrenals with herbals and adrenal glandulars

There are no hard and fast rules here and it really is a case of trial and error. The most useful to try, possibly in combination, are:

- Ashwagandha – start with 1 g (some people take up to 4 g daily)
- Ginseng – use 1-3 g of the root powder
- Bovine adrenal glandular – cortex 150-450 mg
- Pregnenolone 25-100 mg – this is the most upstream of the adrenal hormones, also dubbed the 'memory hormone'. (By being 'upstream' I mean that subsequent hormones are synthesised from it as shown in Figure 4.1: The hormone cascade, courtesy of Dr Linda Gedeon (www.drlindagedeon.com). You can see, for example, DHEA, cortisol, all the sex hormones, aldosterone (a mineralocorticoid) on this cascade, all downstream of pregnenolone. You can also see that cholesterol is the starting point for all)
- DHEA 25-100 mg.

Figure 4.1: The hormone cascade, courtesy of Dr Linda Gedeon (with permission, www.drlindagedeon.com)

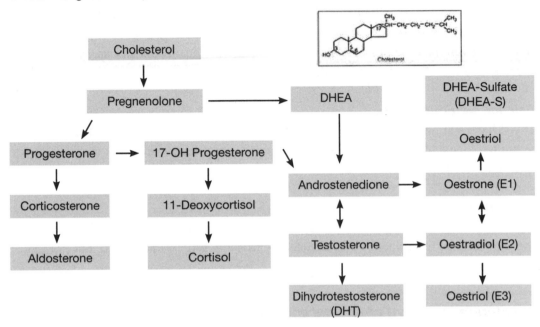

All the above supplements should be taken on rising or split into two doses taken on rising and at midday. This is to mimic the normal diurnal (24-hour) rhythm of adrenal hormones.

Cortisone cream

Cortisol is the hormone that is in most demand and the adrenals make this in preference to all else; consequently, taking hydrocortisone cream 1% 1-2 ml (10-20 mg) by rubbing it into the skin is often remarkably helpful in providing adrenal support. This dose is physiological and so there is no adrenal gland suppression. You can purchase it over the counter.

The risk of suppressing adrenal function

The use of any of the above products in these doses does not suppress adrenal function. The idea is to plug a gap where such exists – to prop up and support whilst the adrenal glands recover. This renders these treatments extremely safe. By contrast, mainstream doctors prescribe adrenal hormones in huge, non-physiological, immune-suppressing doses which switch off endogenous production and cause long-term, life-threatening side effects. The commonest steroid used is prednisolone (*not* to be confused with pregnenolone!). Even the dose of steroids in asthma inhaler medications, nasal sprays and skin creams may be sufficient to cause adrenal suppression.

Salt and water imbalance
If you have symptoms of salt and water imbalance, start with increasing salt and fat in your diet, then add in liquorice 1-5 g of root powder (not the sweet, black stuff otherwise known as 'all sorts'[¶])

Conclusion
Which of the above preparations you use depends on your core temperature readings and the 'how do you feel?' factor. It is, as noted, a 'trial and error' experiment[#], but one that is well worth it.

Monitoring treatment of adrenal and thyroid remedies using core temperature

If all energy delivery mechanisms are working well, we should have an average and stable core temp of 36.7 to 37.3°C (98-99°F). If we do not, then we need to read the next chapter and act accordingly.

[¶]**Historical note:** The story goes that in 1899, a Bassett's sales representative, called Charlie Thompson, whilst visiting a client in Leicester, tripped over and dropped a tray of samples, mixing up all the various sweets. Charlie scrambled to re-arrange them, but the client was intrigued and liked the idea of lots of different sweets mixed up. Soon thereafter, Bassett's began to mass-produce 'allsorts' and they became a successful product.

[#]**Historical note:** The phrase 'trial and error' was, according to WH Thorpe (Professor of Animal Ethology at the University of Cambridge, 1902 – 1986), a term devised by C Lloyd Morgan (British ethologist and psychologist, 1852 – 1936) after having tried out similar phrases such as 'trial and failure' and 'trial and practice'. Under 'Morgan's Canon', animal behaviour should be explained in the simplest possible way – that is, higher mental faculties should only be considered as explanations if lower faculties could not explain a behaviour.

Assess this by using a FIR skin thermometer (very quick and easy) in a warm room (say 20°C (68°F) to check your temperature several times a day. Interpretation must take into account:

- Thyroid hormones are long-acting and 'base load'. The average core temperature reflects thyroid function.
- Adrenal hormones act in seconds, minutes and hours. With perfect matching of energy demand to delivery, the core temperature is remarkably stable. We can use fluctuations of core temperature to assess adrenal function.

If, despite reasonable rest and good doses of adrenal support (as above), there is still marked fluctuation of temperature, this may point to the immune system being active in an attempt to deal with a chronic infection. This can be a useful clue in treating patients with ME (characterised by poor energy delivery *and* chronic inflammation).

These temperature readings allow one to balance up the underactive thyroid and adrenal glands, and in practice we address the two simultaneously as they often co-exist. In essence, the procedure is this:

- If core temperatures fluctuate 'too much' (this will be measured by the actual temperature fluctuations themselves, but also consider the 'how do I feel' factor), then our adrenals are not at their personal optimal function and so we should consider support with one, or more, of the above supplements – herbals, glandulars, pregnenolone, etc.
- If the average core temperature is 'too low' (and this will be measured by the actual temperature – say less than 36.7°C (98°F) – and also consider the 'how do I feel' factor) then the thyroid is not at our personal optimal function and so we should consider support with thyroid glandular (see Chapter 5).
- As noted, we normally do these two things in tandem – they are often inextricably linked.

Read on for more detail and a worked example. We end this chapter with a theatrical note from Craig that carries an important message.

Avoiding your personal 'dangerous corner'

The first stage of adrenal support is to take the pressure off the adrenals, and I think one should not forget that sometimes having fun is a good way of doing this. For me, theatre trips are one of my greatest joys. In fact, the principal tenet of this chapter reminds me of a play by J B Priestley called *Dangerous Corner*, which I had the great pleasure of seeing at the Theatre Royal Windsor, with my wife, Penny, in 2014. The plot can be summarised briefly, and I have done this below, in such a way that there is only a very small spoiler. The choice is yours, dear reader – read this last paragraph in this chapter or turn the page…

There is a gathering of friends at a country retreat and a chance remark by one of the guests leads to a series of incredible revelations. These revelations uncover a tangled web of previously unknown relationships and dark secrets, leading ultimately to devastating consequences. The play ends with a time-slip back to the beginning of the evening at the moment when the chance remark was originally made, and this time it is not made, the secrets remain hidden, and the 'dangerous corner' is thus avoided. The moral here is that we all face 'dangerous corners' in our lives, where things could go one way or the other – we may spin off the road in our sports car at such a dangerous corner.

Now in the case of the adrenals and thyroid, we get early warnings of such a dangerous corner, just like a road signpost and so, unlike the characters in Priestley's play, we can act to avoid falling foul of said impending danger. These early warning signs are the symptoms listed in Chapter 1 and the blood test results from Chapter 2, and also the temperature readings in this chapter and the next. If you recognise these signs, do not ignore them, take the actions as described in this book, and avoid your own personal dangerous corner, with all its attendant devastating consequences.

Chapter 5

How to trial
thyroid glandular (TG)

This chapter shows you how to trial TG, balance up the dose over the long term and manage it with day-by-day tweakings.

All diagnosis starts with hypothesis. In medicine we call this a differential diagnosis. It is confirmed by treatment. That means we embark on a trial and see how this manifests clinically and whether it is confirmed biochemically. Before embarking on such a trial of TG, again check that you have established:
* the PK diet
* vitamin C to bowel tolerance, possibly with Lugol's iodine at night
* the Basic Package (see Groundhog Basic, page 147)
  and, if indicated
* the mitochondrial package of supplements
* the adrenals package – see suggested herbal support and adrenal glandulars in Chapter 4.

Then you need to do blood tests for the level of
* TSH
* free T4
* free T3.

The main reason for checking thyroid hormone levels is to make sure the thyroid is not overactive. This is rare but the last thing one wants is to use thyroid glandular in such a case. The second reason is to see if there is biochemical scope for a trial of thyroid glandular (see Chapter 2).

45

Thyroid glandular (TG)

Hypothyroidism was first recognised in the 1890s and treated then with TG.* It has remained the best treatment for the underactive thyroid. It derives from the whole dried (desiccated) thyroid glands of pigs or cows. Whilst many patients do well on synthetic thyroxin, TG is more physiological since it supplies bio-identical hormones and contains all the iodinated proteins. Importantly TG is a food supplement product and available to all (see Appendix B).

The key to a trial of TG is to start with very low doses and proceed slowly. This is for at least three reasons:

- Thyroid hormones make mitochondria run faster. To achieve this, mitochondria will need all the raw materials described in Chapter 3. They also need time to incorporate them into their biochemistry.
- There is a 'sweet spot' in the level of glandular needed. Thyroid hormones have a long half-life in the body – longer than one day – which means that at any one time the level may reflect several days of treatment. In this event, it is too easy to over-shoot that 'sweet spot' and end up over-dosing.
- Thyroid hormones also determine the number of mitochondria. This makes the difference between a small and a large 'engine'. Guess what? I want to live with a Rolls Royce, not a Mini-Minor!† It takes time to build a bigger engine.

We need to mimic the normal circadian rhythm, with highest levels of thyroid in the morning which then decline as the day progresses. Remember, people who are hypothyroid are often owls, by which I mean they sleep in late and stay up late. Glandular products are best absorbed sublingually (under the tongue) and absorption is

---

Historical note: Readers interested in the history of the use of thyroid glandulars should see the 2011 article by Lindholm and Laurberg, which ' states that: 'Murray published the first account of a human patient with hypothyroidism given substitution with thyroid extract. Clinically, the effect was beyond doubt. The patient lived almost 30 years on thyroid substitution—eventually to die of cardiac failure in 1919.'[1] This patient's life history was recorded by Murray in a 1920 paper, in the *British Medical Journal*.[2]

†**Note from Craig:** My beloved MGB GT may be small in size, but it has a 1.8 litre engine. And it has 'overdrive' so that energy demand can be better matched to energy supply – see https://drmyhill.co.uk/wiki/Craig%27s_MGB_GT.

blocked by caffeine, oestrogen, proton pump inhibitors and statins. Also, minerals such as iron and calcium, and foods that include gluten, dairy and sugar (not permitted on a PK diet) block absorption. You get most 'bang for your buck' by taking them under your tongue and without other supplements. I suggest you keep the pot next to your bed, take a first dose on rising then put your second dose in a pocket so, wherever you happen to be around midday, you can use it then. Having said that, some do perfectly well taking a once-a-day dose on rising.

There are several preparations of glandular available (see Appendix B). Different people are suited by different preparations so there will be an element of trial and eorror but a suggested regime is shown in Table 5.1.

Table 5.1: A suggested schedule for trialling TG

Week	What to take	When (sublingually)	Notes – throughout the trial
1	TG 15 mg procine	1 x capsule on rising	Occasionally measure your core temperature as below (36.7-37.3°C) and pulse rate at rest (70-85 bpm)
2	TG 15 mg porcine	1 x capsule onrising 1 x capsule midday	Occasionally measure blood pressure (BP) (110/60-130/85 mm Hg) Make clinical notes – how do you feel?
3	TG 15 mg porcine	2 x capsules on rising 1 x capsule midday	At this point measure temperature several times a day for 4 days and record as below (Table 5.2)
4	TG 15 mg porcine	2 x capsules on rising 2 x capsules midday	
	OR TG 30 mg porcine	1 x capsule on rising 1 x capsule midday	
5	TG 60 mg porcine	Continue to increase the TG dose every 2 weeks in similar increments until…	…core temperatures, BP and pulse have normalised. Your underactive symptoms are better and there are no symptoms of over-treatment

Table 5.1 (cont'd)

Week	What to take	When (sublingually)	Notes – throughout the trial
7 and there-after		Most need TG 60 mg porcine (TG 65 mg bovine). Assuming a capsule size of 30 mg, then most need 2-6 capsules daily depending on body weight. Typically take per day: up to 9 stone (57 kg): 2–3 up to 12 stone (76 kg): 3–4 up to 15 stone (95 kg): 5 >15 stone (95 kg): 5–6	If you do not feel better at this level, then first review all energy delivery mechanisms. If all interventions are in place, then you must have a hole in the energy bucket; this is so often an infectious hole – see our book *The Infection Game*
			If you lose weight on the PK diet, reduce the number of capsules accordingly

Balancing up the thyroid and the adrenal support

- Do four days of temperature measurements, with at least six a day.
- Calculate the average temperature (all readings for the day divided by the number of readings – this reflects thyroid function) and temperature wobble (i.e. the difference between the lowest reading and the highest in the day – this reflects adrenal function).
- Table 5.2 gives a worked example. All readings should be taken at rest. Allow a few days after the dose change to take these measurements.

Be aware that worsening of symptoms may occur as a result of detox and Herxheimer reactions – see Appendix G. Heat and fever kill microbes so you risk 'allergic or toxic' reactions to dead microbes. If this happens to you, make the changes more slowly as described in see Appendix G.

Table 5.2: Worked example of self-monitoring for thyroid and adrenal function

Week	Daily dose (15 mg capsules)	Temperature through the day (°C)	Average tempera-ture (°C)	Temperature wobble [whilst on] (°C)	Pulse (bpm)	Blood pressure (mm Hg)	How do you feel? Action
1	1	36.1 35.7 35.9 36.5 35.8 35.5	35.8	1.0 on pregnenolone 25 mg	64	112/66	Sluggish Increase pregne-nolone to 50 mg
2	2	35.6 35.9 36.6 36.0 35.8 36.2	35.9	1.0 on pregnenolone 50 mg	66	114/74	Sluggish Increase pregne-nolone to 50 mg
3	3	36.5 36.9,36.6, 36.7 36.5 36.6	36.6	0.4 on pregnenolone 50 mg	66	120/80	
4	4	36.8 37.2 36.9 36.7 36.9 36.8	36.9	0.5 on pregnenolone 50 mg	70	120/72	Stressful week
5	5	37.0 36.9 37.2 36.8 36.6 37.0	36.9	0.7 on pregnenolone 50 mg	80	117/78	Better. Feels like the sweet spot. Stay at this level

Blood tests to monitor progress

Bloods tests give us the coarse tuning. They should never be relied upon entirely. We also need the clinical input of pulse rate, core temperatures, blood pressure and symptoms to fine tune the dose, as shown in Table 5.2. Common errors are shown in Table 5.3.

Table 5.3: Common errors in monitoring thyroid status

What	Why is this a problem?	Notes
Relying solely on TSH levels to monitor the dose	This is only helpful where there is pure primary hypothyroidism	However, this has become the normal way for all doctors to monitor all cases of underactive thyroid
	There is no universal agreement on what the threshold should be and in the UK it is set too high except in pregnancy	In the USA the threshold for prescribing thyroid hormones is a TSH above 3.0 mIU/l. In UK the threshold may be as high as 10.0 mIU/l though the usual threshold used in pregnancy is 1.5 mIU/l I like to see the TSH below 1.5 mIU/l in all patients
	With pituitary insufficiency (or secondary hypothyroidism) expect to see TSH suppressed e.g. <0.01 mIU/l	I suspect this is more common where there is adrenal fatigue
	I like to see the TSH below 1.5 mIU/l	This is the usual threshold used in pregnancy. The IQ of the baby is inversely proportionate to the TSH of the mother[3]
Free T4 My range is 12-24pmoll Some NHS ranges are 7-14pmol/l	The references ranges have changed markedly in my clinical career. This is because ref ranges are based on "normal" people and now that hypothyroidism is so common the range has fallen. So, the goalposts have been moved!	
	Some do not feel well until the fT4 is at 30pmol/l. Not my words but those of Professor Sir Anthony Toft who wrote "The British Medical Association Guide to Treating Hypothyroidism" See https://www.drmyhill.co.uk/wiki/Thyroid_disease_-_how_to_persuade_your_GP_to_diagnose_and_treat for a book review	
Free T3 3.2-6.8	If low this points to under-dosing If high, it may be that the test was taken too soon after dosing and taking the temperature. T3 is short acting. Allow at least 6 hours between.	

Underactive thyroid in pregnancy is a particular concern because of the effect on the growing child. In their 2004 study 'Attention Deficit and Hyperactivity Disorders in the Offspring of Mothers Exposed to Mild-Moderate Iodine Deficiency', Vermiglio et al, concluded that children's total IQ (combination of 'performal' IQ and verbal IQ) was inversely correlated to the mother's TSH at mid-term, so that the lower the TSH, the higher the total IQ. This result was significant at 99.9% confidence levels.[3]

There you have it – the immediate, practical nitty gritty of how to do it. But you have not finished yet!

It is my experience that there are often several reasons for the thyroid to be under-active (see Chapter 6). If these are all addressed as best you can, then the need for glandulars may diminish. An obvious factor is weight loss – large people need larger doses than small people and a good PK diet makes it so much easier to lose weight and get fit. Improving nutrition and reducing the toxic load together reduce the biochemical friction. Putting the body into a low state of inflammation may be of further help. Read on![‡] [Doof Doof!]

[‡]**Postscript from Craig:** The reader may have noticed the repetition of 'Read on' commands at the end of chapters? I am reminded of the soap, *Eastenders*, and its famous cliff-hanger moments at the end of episodes, which are always denoted by the 'Doof Doof' of the first bar of the music, as the camera zooms in on the character facing impending doom, or whatever. There is even a website listing the fans' favourite 'Doof Doof' moments https://eastenders.fandom.com/wiki/Doof_Doofs%27). Yes, I do watch *Eastenders*. I claim exemption from ridicule via Oscar Wilde (1854 – 1900): 'I adore simple pleasures. They are the last refuge of the complex.'

Part II

The theory

Chapter 6

How and why we become hypothyroid:
The mechanisms

Hypothyroidism is common because of the deficiencies and toxicities of Western life. It is likely to arise for several such reasons and, in consequence, patients that I see often have more than one type of hypothyroidism. This is obvious from Table 6.1.

Table 6.1: Causes of hypothyroidism

Type	Mechanism/Example medical papers where relevant	How to fix it
Primary hypothy-roidism – when the thyroid is malfunctioning	The thyroid does not have the raw materials to make thyroid hormones. The commonest deficiency is of iodine (see Chapter 13) but many other nutrients are involved[1]	Apply Groundhog Basic (Appendix D)
	OR The thyroid has been destroyed by autoimmunity. This may be switched on by viral infection, including Epstien Barr (EBV), hepatitis A, B and C, parvovirus B19, herpes I and II, HTLV and SARS Covid-2[2, 3, 4, 5, 6]	Once destroyed you cannot regrow new thyroid tissue – it is thyroid support for life as the only solution
	We are seeing epidemics of auto-immunity due to vaccination, vitamin D deficiency and Western pro-inflammatory diets (sugar and refined carbs, gluten and dairy products) – see studies referenced in Chapter 2	Avoid vaccination – look after the immune system with Groundhog regimes (Appendix D) PK diet for life (Appendix C) Vitamin D 10,000 iu daily for life

Table 6.1 (cont'd)

Type	Mechanism/Example medical papers where relevant	How to fix it
	Direct damage by viral or bacterial infection (thyroiditis). This may present with an acute febrile illness, pain and swelling of the thyroid. Offending microbes include mumps, coxsackie A and B, ECHO, possibly CMV, measles, chickenpox, rubella, adenovirus, influenza and SARS Covid-2[7, 8]	Some people are genetically predisposed to this with tissue type HLA B35[14]
	The thyroid has been poisoned by halides (fluoride, bromide),[12, 13] heavy metals (mercury, lead),[9, 10, 11] sex hormones (Pill and HRT – see Chapter 1), prescription drugs (lithium, amiodarone) and/or perhaps electromagnetic radiation	See Chapter 9
	Damage by physical injury, e.g. whiplash	Once destroyed you cannot regrow new thyroid tissue – it is thyroid support for life
	Thyroiditis may be accompanied by thyrotoxicosis (De Quervain's)	
	Often results from the over-treatment of thyrotoxicosis with carbimazole, radiation or surgery (see Chapter 13)[15]	Following any such treatment, you must very closely monitor your thyroid status with blood tests and clinical checks (pulse, core temperature, blood pressure and symptoms)
T3 hypothy-roidism	When the thyroid cannot convert inactive T4 to the active T3 because of deficiency[16] or	Groundhog Basic – supplies iron, selenium, zinc, magnesium and vitamin D
	because of blocking[17, 18, 19, 20, 21, 22, 23]	Detox regimes – see Appendix F
Secondary hypothy-roidism	The pituitary is under-active due to deficiency or poisoning e.g. by organo-phosphate pesticides.[24] Or by drugs: steroids, dopamine agonists (Parkinson's disease), cancer chemotherapy	Groundhog Basic – see Appendix D Detox regimes – see Appendix F

	The pituitary is damaged due to acute blood loss or severe drop in blood pressure, due to stroke (e.g. clotting post covid-19 vaccination) or bleeding.[25] This is important and a common cause of post -stroke fatigue	Damage following a major haemorrhage during childbirth is called Sheehan syndrome[27]
	The pituitary is damaged due to head injury – typically a fracture of the base of the skull[25]	Usually thyroid hormones for life
	Pituitary tumour	Usually thyroid hormones for life
Thyroid hormone receptor resistance	The circulating thyroid hormones are blocked or inhibited by • reverse T3 • prescription drugs such as beta blockers • toxins from the fermenting gut • exogenous toxins • genetic link[26]	Detox regimes – see Appendix F

Table 6.1 is helpful to determine root causes, which sometimes can be reversed (see Appendix F: Detoxing). However, almost regardless of the mechanism, correction can be achieved with the judicious use of thyroid glandulars as described in Chapters 1 to 5.

The evidence: Studies

Study 1: Iodine deficiency

In 'The Iodine Deficiency Disorders Creswell and Zimmermann gave details, for example, in Table 2, of the links between iodine deficiency and hypothyroidism.[1]

Study 2: Infection and autoimmunity

In 'Covid-19 and autoimmunity', Ehrenfeld et al stated that: 'The most prominent patho-genic viruses which have been proposed in the triggering and initiation of autoimmune diseases include Parvovirus B19, Epstein-Barr-virus (EBV), Cytomegalovirus (CMV), Herpes virus-6, HTLV-1, Hepatitis A and C virus, and Rubella virus.'[2] This comprehensive study is complete with full referencing of 143 further medical papers, specifically mentioning Hashimoto thyroiditis and autoimmune hepatitis and with a full discussion of Covid-19 and autoimmune disorders, including autoimmune hypothyroidism.

Study 3: Epstein-Barr virus (EBV) and autoimmunity

In their 2015 paper, 'The role of Epstein-Barr virus infection in the development of autoimmune thyroid diseases', Janegova et al reported that 81% of Hashimoto's thyroiditis cases and 63% of Graves' disease cases that they examined had EBV proteins evident in the thyroid gland and therefore proposed an aetiological role for EBV in the development of these autoimmune thyroid diseases.[3]

Study 4: Covid and underactive thyroid

In 2021 Ruggeri et al, in their paper 'SARS-COV-2-related immune-inflammatory thyroid disorders: facts and perspectives', stated that: 'COVID-19-related thyroid disorders include destructive thyroiditis and onset or relapse of autoimmune thyroid disorders, leading to a broad spectrum of thyroid dysfunction ranging from thyrotoxicosis to hypothyroidism.'[4]

Study 5: Viral hepatitis and autoimmunity

In 1996, Catapani et al, in the *BMJ* discussed the fact that cases where hepatitis B is associated with autoimmune thyroid diseases are far fewer than with hepatitis C but that this does not necessarily exclude causal links.[5]

Study 6: Hepatitis C and autoimmune thyroid disorders

In their 2016 paper, 'Hepatitis C virus infection and thyroid autoimmune disorders: A model of interactions between the host and the environment',Pastore et al stated that: 'Autoimmune thyroid diseases are common in HCV infected patients.'[6]

Studies 7 and 8: Infection and autoimmune thyroiditis

In their 2021 paper, 'The association of subacute thyroiditis with COVID-19: A systematic review', Rehman et alreferenced studies showing links between all the pathogens listed below and thyroiditis, stating that: '…multiple viruses have been implicated as a trigger for subacute thyroiditis since then. Some of them include mumps, measles, rubella, influenza, coxsackie, adenovirus, varicella zoster virus, cytomegalovirus, Epstein-Barr virus, hepatitis E, and HIV….'[7] They also referenced 13 further studies of which they said: 'The increasing evidence of SAT during or after the COVID-19 infection has been reported in various published cases ….'

This supports the comprehensive 2009 study by Desailloud and Hober who presented epidemiological and virological evidence, along with case reports, showing '…evidence of the presence of viruses or their components in the organ… … for retroviruses (HFV) and mumps in subacute thyroiditis, for retroviruses (HTLV-1, HFV, HIV and SV40) in Graves's disease and for HTLV-1, enterovirus, rubella, mumps virus, HSV, EBV and parvovirus in Hashimoto's thyroiditis'.[8]

Studies 9-11: Heavy metals and thyroid disorders

Studies linking hypothyroidism with heavy metal toxicity include:
   a. For lead, Pekcici et al stated in their 2010 paper: 'Clinicians should be aware of the potential hazardous effects of lead on the thyroid, especially in patients who have been occupationally exposed to lead.'[9]
   b. For mercury, Urinyova et al state in their 2012 paper: 'low-level exposure to Hg [mercury] can affect thyroid hormone status during prenatal and early postnatal exposure depending on the form of Hg, gender, ethnicity, lifestyle, or socioeconomic status (dental amalgam fillings).'[10]
   c. For cadmium, Chen et al in their 2013 paper stated: 'Our analysis suggests … a positive association between Cd [cadmium] exposure and thyroid hormones in adults.'[11]

Studies 12 and 13: Bromide poisoning and thyroid problems

In his chapter in the online publication *Endotext*, David Sarne noted that both fluorine and bromine block iodide transport into the thyroid gland and that bromine is concentrated by the thyroid and interferes with thyroidal uptake in animals and humans, possibly by competitive inhibition of iodide transport into the gland.[12] Note that fluorides are used routinely in dental treatments, toothpastes and increasingly in mains water. Bromides are used as fire retardants in soft furnishings – which explains why all Sarah's sofas and chairs are ancient!

Kim Maskall stated in her 2018 article on the *Pledging Change* website: 'Studies show that the chemicals used in flame retardants in furnishings which can migrate and settle in dust in our homes, have shown up in breast milk, babies and toddlers as well. What is known and very alarming is that these levels are known to lower the IQ and can slow down brain development in early years.'[13]

Study 14 : SAT and thyroid problems

In their 2004 paper, 'Familial occurrence of subacute thyroiditis associated with human leukocyte antigen-B35', Kramer et al described a case report of the second familial incidence and largest family reported so far with occurrence of SAT in association with HLA-B35.[14]

Study 15: Treatment for thyrotoxicosis and long-term underactive thyroid

In their 2021 paper 'Thyrotoxicosis', Blick et al stated that: 'Hypothyroidism usually occurs within 6 to 12 months [of radioiodine therapy]' and that: 'Total or partial thyroidectomy is a rapid and effective method of treating thyrotoxicosis. However, it is invasive and expensive, and causes permanent hypothyroidism, requiring levothyroxine treatment.'[15]

Study 16: Vitamins. Minerals and thyroid status

In their 2020 paper, 'Thyroid-gut-axis: How does the microbiota influence thyroid function?', Knezevic et al stated that: 'Iodine, iron, and copper are crucial for thyroid hormone synthesis, selenium and zinc are needed for converting T4 to T3, and vitamin D assists in regulating the immune response.'[16]

Studies 17-23: Toxins and underactive thyroid

- In the report 'Environmental toxins and their role in thyroid diseases', the Mindd Foundation listed the following references showing that heavy metals, household toxins, industrial chemicals and agricultural agents block thyroid function.[17]
- Acconcia et al 2015: 'Molecular mechanisms of action of BPA.'[18]
- Bajaj et al, 2016. 'Various possible toxicants involved in thyroid dysfunction: A review.'[19]
- Brent, 2010. 'Environmental exposures and autoimmune thyroid disease.'[20]
- Ferrari et al, 2017. 'Environmental issues in thyroid diseases.'[21]
- Konieczna et al, 2015. 'Health risk exposure to Bisphenol A (BPA).'[22]
- Vojdani, 2014. 'A potential link between environmental triggers and autoimmunity.'[23]

Study 24: Organophosphates and pituitary damage

In 2015, Dutta et al reported that 14 patient with acute organophosphate poisoning were shown to have hormonal alterations similar to 'sick euhormonal syndrome' three months after the initial poisoning.[24]

Study 25: Brain injury and pituitary dysfunction

In their 2018 paper 'Pituitary dysfunction and association with fatigue in stroke and other acute brain injury', Booij et al stated that following stroke and other acquired brain injury data there is a high prevalence of pituitary dysfunction.[25]

Study 26: Resistance to thyroid hormone due to receptor mutations

In their 2017 paper 'A clinician's guide to understanding resistance to thyroid hormone due to receptor mutations in the TRα and TRβ isoforms', Singh and Yen reviewed causes of thyroid resistance.[26]

Study 27: National Organization for Rare Diseases (Nord)[27]

Light relief – Colouring maps

The authors are again aware that those who have followed the links to the studies in this chapter will need some light relief. Craig therefore gives you a maths problem! It was posed thus: in the early 1850s the question was asked, 'What is the minimum number of colours required to colour ANY map so that no two adjacent regions (i.e. with a common boundary segment) are of the same colour.

The answer is four and, like all good mathematics, is perhaps somewhat surprising. You might, if you are like me when I was first told this, go off and try to draw a map that needed five colours? Anyway, you can see more here: https://en.wikipedia.org/wiki/Four_color_theorem

Just to add, the proof of this theorem was computer-assisted and cannot be proven by 'pen and paper' by a human. This proof is therefore called a 'non-surveyable proof' by the philosophers of mathematics, (https://en.wikipedia.org/wiki/Non-surveyable_proof) so, initially, it was not accepted by all mathematicians. However, the proof has gained wide acceptance, although some doubters remain….

Chapter 7

What happens if the diagnosis of hypothyroidism is missed?

The short answer to this question is 'Chronic fatigue syndrome, disease, degeneration and premature death'. Simple as that. This chapter explains why.

The thyroid is centrally involved in energy delivery mechanisms and all cells in the body are impacted by such. If cells go slow, organs go slow. Hypothyroidism is associated with all organ failures, any of which may lead to death. Missing the diagnosis and undertreating therefore has very serious consequences. More reasons to do it yourself. Incentivise yourself by a quick look at the nasties listed in Table 7.1.

Table 7.1: The short-term and long-term results of slow energy delivery due to underactive thyroid

Slow energy delivery to:	Short term results in:	Long term results in:
- The muscles of the body	Weakness and inability to get fit	Chronic fatigue syndrome (and, if the immune system is involved too – see below – then myalgic encephalitis). Myxoedema coma
- The brain	Foggy brain, poor short-term memory	Myxoedema madness Dementia
	You look miserable The face is a mirror of the brain	You appear prematurely aged
- The sense organs	Deteriorating vision, hearing, smell, taste and touch	Blindness, deafness, anosmia, numbness

Table 7.1 (cont'd)

Slow energy delivery to:	Short term results in:	Long term results in:
- Ion pumps in cell membranes	Fluid leaks out of cells – puffy face, puffy ankles	Tissue swelling creates pressure on nerves – nerve compression syndromes such as carpal tunnel
- The immune system	Tendency to pick up all the infections doing the rounds	Overwhelming infection and possible death, typically from pneumonia. All the downstream effects of chronic infections e.g., cancer, dementia – see our book *The Infection Game*
- ...also responsible for healing and repair	We wear out our bodies with use and heal and repair with rest. Get the balance wrong and we degenerate	Connective tissue loss, with degeneration of joint muscle and tendon, gut lining, blood vessels, skin, hair, nails and bone (osteoporosis)
- The bone marrow	Poor immunity as above. Anaemia	Risk of overwhelming infection as above. Worsening anaemia
	Poor cancer surveillance	Increased risk of cancer
- The heart	Weakness and inability to get fit	Heart failure
- The liver	Worsening ability to clear toxins (may manifest with drug or alcohol intolerance)	Liver failure
- The kidneys	Early disease may be seen on blood tests, with rising creatinine	Kidney failure
- The hormone-producing glands	Deficiency syndromes	Infertility
- The lungs	Thankfully these are powered for the business of extreme exercise so poor energy delivery is rarely pathological	
- The organs of reproduction	Loss of libido – Nature's way of telling us we do not have the reserves for the energy intensive business of reproduction	Infertility

Bear all the possible consequences in mind because your doctor will only tell you of the risks of taking thyroid hormones, *not* of the risks of *not* taking them. S/he will tell you that you are overdosing because the only blood test they rely on to assess the dose level is the TSH, as described in Chapter 1. S/he forgets, or does not know, that most are hypothyroid for many possible reasons and the TSH is often misleading. Read on! [Doof Doof!]

Perhaps more light relief is needed? See next. But please, dear reader, do not forget the message of this chapter – missing a diagnosis of hypothyroidism can be fatal.

Light relief – That number 1089, by Craig

1. Take any three-digit number, where the first and last digits differ by more than one.
2. Reverse the number to produce a new one.
3. Then subtract the smaller number from the larger number, producing another new number.
4. If you reverse this new number and this time add the two, the result will *always* be 1089.

For example…
1. …if we begin with 452…
2. Reversed we get 254.
3. Taking the smaller from the larger, we get $452 - 254 = 198$.
4. If we reverse this number and then add the two, we get $891 + 198 = 1089$.

Impress your friends and family!

Most mathematicians can pinpoint a 'moment' when they got hooked by mathematics. For me, it was when someone told me that if you divide the circumference of any (*any!*) circle by its diameter, you always (*always!*) get the same number – pi, π. I just had to know more! And even now, I 'do' mathematics nearly every day of my life.

For one of my tutors, Dave Acheson, that 'moment' concerned the number 1089. He has written a book about it – *1089 and All That* and this YouTube shows Dave at his best discussing 1089 and another surprise in mathematics: www.youtube.com/watch?v=BJ7_fFABc9s&t=9s. Dave's tutorials were the most memorable of all – they consisted of drinking tea, listening to his guitar playing, and of course doing maths, not all of which related to the actual modules we were meant to be studying. It is my honour and privilege to have been his tutee. If I may persist, watch Dave solve a geometry/road-building problem with soap bubbles here: www.youtube.com/watch?v=_O-z_slpzzw&t=136s

Chapter 8

Thyroid myths
How your doctor will discourage you

These days, it seems, doctors have increasingly high levels of 'negative capability'. This term was first used by Romantic poet John Keats in 1817 to explain the capacity of the greatest writers (particularly Shakespeare) to pursue a vision of artistic beauty even when it leads them into intellectual confusion and uncertainty. The term is now used to describe the ability to perceive and recognise great 'truths' without the need for consecutive reasoning. Negative capability is fantastic if you are a Romantic poet or great writer, but it has no place in medicine.

So, doctors, using their full powers of negative capability, will tell you that, if you take thyroid glandular 'You will get atrial fibrillation. You will get osteoporosis'.

No! This is only a risk with chronic over-dosing, and your job, as described in Chapter 5, is to find that 'sweet spot'* of perfect control. Indeed, having an underactive thyroid is also a risk factor for heart disease and osteoporosis. So, let us employ belt and braces – what more can be done to prevent such problems?

Doctors love single symptoms and simple solutions. Both heart disease and osteoporosis have many causes which collectively may result in disease. Of course, the Groundhog regimes are highly protective against these conditions, but people come to me too late, with established problems, so let's do it all.

*Footnote: The origin of the phrase 'sweet spot' is almost definitely from sports, for example, where there is a 'sweet spot' on the surface of a racquet that gives the most power for the least effort. Traditionally golfers have laid claim to its first use in *The New York Times* of 16 March 1957, with the headline, 'Trigonometry Finds "Sweet Spot" for the Golf Club to Meet the Ball'. Whatever the truth, the phrase describes very well what we are after – the minimum dose required to achieve the desired effect.

Atrial fibrillation

Atrial fibrillation (AF) is an increasingly common problem; in the UK its prevalence is about 2.5%. It is easy to diagnose – the pulse becomes completely irregular. What happens in atrial fibrillation is that the pacemaker of the heart ceases to function properly so that the two top chambers of the heart – namely, the left and right atria – instead of contracting in an organised, rhythmical fashion simply wobble about in an uncoordinated way.

We have to ask why the pacemaker is malfunctioning. Yes, we know this is a complication of both an overactive and an underactive thyroid but there are other causes as well, listed in Table 8.1.

Table 8.1: Causes of atrial fibrillation (AF)

Causes of AF	Why	Action
The natural pacemaker of the heart does not have the energy to work	Poor blood supply due to arterial disease or anaemia	Angiogram to diagnose Measure homocysteine[1] Apply Groundhog Chronic – Appendix D
	Poor energy delivery mechanisms	Read the rest of this book! Groundhog Chronic – Appendix D
The electrical conduction system within the heart malfunctions	Magnesium deficiency	Magnesium 300 mg, and vitamin D 10,000 iu for its absorption. (By the way, this usually cures ventricular ectopics, the commonest cardiac dysrhythmia) – see the open-access paper by DiNicolantonio et al (2018) which includes: '…a study in postmenopausal women found that a low-magnesium diet (approximately 100 mg/day) can induce atrial fibrillation' And 'Magnesium therapy may be useful in the treatment of refractory ventricular tachycardia, ventricular fibrillation, multifocal atrial tachycardia, atrial fibrillation and supraventricular tachycardia'[2]

Causes of AF	Why	Action
	Iodine deficiency	See Chapter 13
	Poisoning by toxic metals	See Chapter 6 and 9
	Poisoning by pesticides	See Chapter 6 and 9
	Too much stimulation by caffeine, chocolate or adrenalin produced in response to stress for an already sick heart	Avoid
		Much more detail in our book *Ecological Medicine*

Osteoporosis

Table 8.2: The causes of osteoporosis

Causes of osteoporosis	Why	Action
Metabolic syndrome from a 'standard Western diet' – that is, sugar, carbs and junk food	All the reasons detailed below and inflammation	PK diet – fuel the body with fat and fibre, not sugar and starch
Micronutrient deficiency	Calcium, magnesium, boron, phosphorus, zinc, silica and strontium essential for bone structure	Take the basic package of supplements as in Groundhog Basic (Appendix D). Bone broth is full of the raw materials for making bone
Vitamin D deficiency	Necessary to absorb calcium and magnesium and ensure their deposition in bone	We all need 10,000 iu daily Do not overdo calcium – see below

Table 8.2 (cont'd)

Causes of osteoporosis	Why	Action
Vitamin K deficiency	This comes from green vegetables and the fermentation of fibre by friendly microbes in the lower gut	Vitamin K1 is synthesised in the large bowel by friendly bacteria fermenting fibre. Vitamin K2 is present in animal products and fermented foods. A good PK diet prevents deficiency. If your diet is not fully PK, take vitamin K1 1 mg and K2 1 mg daily
Too much calcium Dairy products increase the risk of osteoporosis	Calcium and magnesium compete for absorption. Too much calcium blocks magnesium absorption	Avoid dairy products (PK diet) - our physiological requirement ratio for calcium to magnesium is about 2:1. In dairy products the ratio is 10:1, so consuming dairy products will induce a magnesium deficiency. Do not take high-dose calcium supplements Ad-cal (the chewable tablets) do not work for osteoporosis – they contain far too much calcium and insufficient vitamin D. Guzzling these and dairy products is guaranteed to worsen osteoporosis[3] See this open-access paper by Michaëlsson et al (2014) which states that: 'High milk intake was associated with higher mortality in one cohort of women and in another cohort of men, and with higher fracture incidence in women'
Malabsorption – you need an acid stomach to absorb minerals	A common cause of this are proton pump inhibitors, which reduce stomach acid and so cause digestion and absorption issues. The upper fermenting gut malabsorbs	Do a PK diet – then you will not need PPIs or other acid blockers
Lack of exercise	Changing physical forces through bone stimulates micro-electrical currents (the piezo-electric effect) which drive bone formation. Astronauts in space get rapid onset osteoporosis!	Weight-bearing exercise works best to generate the necessary forces through bone. Interested readers should see Singh et al (2014) for more[4]

Treatment and prevention of osteoporosis

First diagnose. I do not like conventional bone density scans which involve high doses of radiation. Ultrasound bone density testing is accurate, completely safe and can be repeated regularly until you know you have put together the necessary package to prevent and/or reverse osteoporosis. Many osteopaths and chiropractors offer this scan. But do not wait for a scan; get on and do all the above, possibly adding in **strontium**.

Strontium is to bone what carbon is to iron – it turns it into steel. There are fabulous studies (see Dean et al (2004),[5] who reference a further 10 studies concerning strontium and osteoporosis.) clearly showing the efficacy of natural strontium 300 mg daily in reversing osteoporosis. Big Pharma rushed to jump on this effective remedy, but of course natural strontium cannot be patented. Big Pharma used an unnatural salt – namely, strontium ranelate – and, to make it palatable, mixed it with aspartame, and therein lies the rub. This unnatural concoction, Protelos, caused an increased risk of thromboembolism, fell out of favour and was discontinued, effective August 2017, with the statement: 'Licensed for the treatment of severe osteoporosis it has been the subject of several safety alerts over the years including life-threatening allergic reactions, venous thromboembolism and increased risk of heart problems. The manufacturer has taken a strategic decision, for commercial reasons, to withdraw the product.'[6]

Don't you just love that the reasons for discontinuation were 'commercial' rather than that it was 'life-threatening'. As always with Big Pharma, follow the money!

By contrast, natural strontium has no such serious side effects. It is safe and inexpensive. However, be aware you need a non-fermenting gut to absorb strontium… yep! It is back to Groundhogs.

Chapter 9

How we starve, destroy and poison the thyroid gland

The overriding message of this chapter is that prevention is better than cure.* For this purpose:

- Don't starve your thyroid by denying it the essential micronutrients it needs.
- Don't switch on autoimmunity and thereby destroy your thyroid.
- Don't poison your thyroid with a multitude of toxins.

It is far harder to 'sort' these problems after the event than to avoid them in the first place.

How we starve the thyroid gland

We begin here with an historical aside to illustrate the importance of getting the balance right. Brilliant German mathematician, Kurt Gödel (1906 – 1978), was famed for his Incompleteness Theorems, which formalised the limitations on what is mathematically provable. However, after the assassination of his close friend Moritz Schlick (German philosopher, 1882 – 1936) by one of his own students, Gödel became paranoid about being poisoned. This fear became so strong that, in later years, he only ate food prepared by his wife, Adele, and when she was hospitalised for a few months after a stroke, Gödel refused to eat and died of starvation in 1978. We have to eat, yet not poison ourselves.

*Footnote: The phrase 'Prevention is better than cure' is most often attributed to Desiderius Erasmus (1466 – 1536). Erasmus was a Dutch philosopher, humanist and theologian. We have tried here, and in all our other books, to follow his advice regarding learning: 'A constant element of enjoyment must be mingled with our studies…'.

This is entirely possible, but something which the great Gödel seemed not to be able to accomplish on his own. See below for how to do it.

Micronutrient deficiency is the single greatest cause, spearheaded by iodine. Iodine deficiency is pandemic, and the risible UK government-recommended daily amount of 150 mcg is far too low for optimum health (see Chapter 13). Anyone with any thyroid issue should have, over and above Groundhog Basic (which supplies 1 mg, or 1000 mcg – see page 147), an additional 50 mg (that is, 3 drops daily of Lugol's 15% iodine). Iodine is one of my favourite multitasking tools (again see Chapter 13).

Other essential minerals for the thyroid include selenium (200 mcg daily), iron (15 mg) and zinc (30 mg), all included in Groundhog Basic (Appendix D). Of course, one needs a non-fermenting gut for optimum absorption, so yes, it's that PK diet too. To paraphrase O'Kane et al (2018), thyroid hormones need proteins, enzymes and iodine for their normal metabolism, and said metabolism is also affected by other micronutrients, such as selenium, zinc, iron and vitamin A.[1]

How we destroy the thyroid gland

Autoimmunity now afflicts 20% of Westerners and the commonest target organ is the thyroid (largely underactive as a result of this attack, and a few overactive). The American Thyroid Association has said: 'Anti-thyroid antibodies are present in up to 20% of the US population,'[2] and a 2020 paper in the journal *Cureus* concluded that '….autoimmune diseases… affect 20% of the entirety of the human population…'.[3]

If you think of your immune system as your standing army whose primary function is to fight off invaders, autoimmunity is civil war. Civil war may start with an attack on the thyroid but could progress to other nasties such as rheumatoid arthritis, type I diabetes, multiple sclerosis, pernicious anaemia and/or another 100+ possibilities. Having one autoimmune disease greatly increases the risk of others.[4]

Autoimmunity is easy to switch on but difficult, perhaps impossible, to switch off. Prevention, as we have already said, is better than cure. So what are the risk factors and how do we avoid them? Table 9.1 shows the main ones.

Table 9.1: The major risk factors for autoimmunity

What	Why	How to avoid
Vaccination		
(see Chapters 1 and 6)	These are designed to switch on the immune system, hopefully just to the targeted microbe, but may switch on generalised inflammation including autoimmunity	Look after the immune system. Nutritional interventions are of proven efficacy. We know from the worldwide covid experiment that PK diet together with vitamins C and D is far superior at preventing serious illness and death than are vaccinations – see www.nhs-corona-doctors-on-the-frontline.com. Click on the 'More' tab for studies showing the efficacy of nutritional interventions with respect to covid
Poor immune function with viral infection (see Chapter 6)	Many autoimmune conditions have an infectious driver. My most hated virus, Epstein Barr ('glandular fever' or 'mono'), afflicts 90% at some stage of life; it is associated with at least 33 different autoimmune conditions[†]	As above. At the first hint of any infection further assist the immune system with Groundhog Acute – see Appendix D. Prevent those infections becoming chronic (which drives many cases of myalgic encephalitis – ME/CFS)
Vitamin D deficiency (See Chapter 1)	Vitamin D is the most important anti-inflammatory. It evolved to prevent inflammation in the skin, and so it is produced there, in high concentrations, through the action of sunlight on cholesterol. This partly explains why incidence of autoimmunity increases with distance from the equator. To quote Schwalfenberg (2012): 'Evidence shows that MS correlates positively with higher latitude, with latitudes >37.5 degrees from the equator having significantly higher rates of MS'[5]	I have never seen adequate blood levels of vitamin D in people not taking supplements. We all need 10,000 iu daily, proportionately less for children. This is roughly equivalent to an hour of UK summer midday sunshine falling directly on full body skin

[†]**Footnote:** For the role of Epstein Barr virus in autoimmune diseases see the study by Janegova in Chapter 6 (reference 3), regarding autoimmune thyroid diseases, and as further examples see studies by Draborg et al (2013), Bagert (2009) and Hjalgrim et al (2007).[8, 9, 10]

Table 9.1 (cont'd)

What	Why	How to avoid
The Pill and HRT (see Chapter 1 – 'Being female')	These artificial hormones dysregulate the immune system and are immunosuppressive, allowing viruses to prevail	The Pill and HRT are dangerous medicine. Ironically they are often used to treat the very symptoms of hypothyroidism – see Chapter 11
Diet: • Allergy, especially to gluten and dairy (see Chapter 2)	Allergy and autoimmunity are both immunological errors. If autoimmunity is civil war, allergy is racism – the attacking of harmless visitors	The PK diet is dairy and gluten free
• Sugar	Sugar is directly pro-inflammatory	The PK diet is low in sugar
• Carbohydrates	These feed the upper fermenting gut. Microbes flourish, spill over into the bloodstream and drive inflammation at distal sites. This is called molecular mimicry and that too drives auto-immunity[‡]	The PK diet is low in carbohydrate
• Friendly gut fermenters	The gut microbiome is an essential part of immune programming	The PK diet is high in fibre and involves eating seasonally. A wide variety of food results in a diverse and therefore healthy microbiome
Silicone implants	Silicones 'bleed' from implants to cause ASIA syndrome (autoimmune/inflammatory syndrome by adjuvants)[6, 7]	Explanting of silicone implants helps to reverse the pathology. Prevention is better than cure – vanity is a killer!
Toxic metals: lead, mercury, aluminium, nickel, arsenic, silver, gold etc (see Chapter 6)	These are immuno-toxic – that is, they also act as immune adjuvants to switch on inflammation. (They are also toxic in their own right)	Avoid! The commonest sources are metals in vaccines, dental metals (mercury, nickel, gold, platinum etc) jewellery and piercings. See below for tests and treatment
Moulds and mycotoxins	These may have direct toxicity and perhaps immune effects[§]	Avoid! Reduce the endogenous load in the gut with the PK diet, in the airways and perineum using an iodine saltpipe and iodine oil. (See our book *The Infection Game*)

How we poison the thyroid

The Ancients knew about poisons and tried to avoid them where they could, though that must have been difficult if you happened to be a courtier to Cleopatra VII of Egypt! For example, in his treatise *On Architecture* (VIII.6.1ff), Vitruvius (c. 80 – 70 BC to after c.15 BC, Roman Engineer and Architect) wrote of his preference for earthen water pipes over lead ones:

> *Water conducted through earthen pipes is more wholesome than that through lead; indeed, that conveyed in lead must be injurious, because from it, white lead [sic PbCO3, lead carbonate] is obtained, and this is said to be injurious to the human system. Hence, if what is generated from it is pernicious, there can be no doubt that itself cannot be a wholesome body. This may be verified by observing the workers in lead, who are of a pallid colour...*

Consequently, Vitruvius never used lead water pipes in his buildings. Good for him, but we are not so lucky these days.

‡**Footnote:** The idea here is that the immune system reacts to an antigen, such as a food or microbe, in the gut. Through pure chance this antigen is the same shape as a cell type in the body. Autoimmunity is switched on because the body 'sees' the cell type as an antigen. Perhaps the best example is ankylosing spondylitis. In this condition, there is molecular mimicry between *klebsiella* bacteria in the gut and the spinal ligaments of people who are HLA B27 positive. So, in essence, the body makes antibodies against *klebsiella* bacteria in the gut and then these antibodies cross-react with spinal ligaments and cause the condition of ankylosing spondylitis.[11]

§**Footnote:** Studies on mould and its effect on the thyroid are in their infancy, but the interested reader is referred to papers by Winzelberg et al (1979), Rotter et al (1994 – includes size of thyroid being reduced) and Wentz (2019).[12,13,14]

Table 9.2: Substances that poison the thyroid

What	Why	How to avoid
The Pill and HRT	These cause nutritional deficiencies – see Palmery et al (2013)[15] who conclude that nutrient depletions occur in folic acid, vitamins B2, B6, B12, vitamin C and E and the minerals magnesium, selenium and zinc when taking the Pill	Avoid taking the Pill and/or HRT
Halides: fluoride and bromides	Biochemically these molecules are very similar to iodine. Iodine deficiency is pandemic and in its absence, the thyroid will grab something similar	Make sure you have plenty of iodine – take Lugol's iodine 15% 3 drops daily (see Chapter 13). Avoid fluoride in water, toothpaste and dental treatments
		Avoid bromides. The main source is polybrominated biphenyls used as fire retardants in soft furnishings. Hang on to those ancient sofas and armchairs!
Toxic metals: lead, mercury, aluminium, nickel, arsenic, silver, gold etc	These inhibit thyroid biochemistry – see Chapter 6	Avoid – the commonest sources are metals in vaccines, dental metals (mercury, nickel, gold, platinum etc), jewellery and piercings, and still lead from old lead pipes. (See below for tests and treatment)
Radiation	The commonest radioactive nucleotide from bombs and industry is iodine 131. The Nevada nuclear tests conducted between 1951 and 1962 killed 11,000 Americans through thyroid cancer. Chernobyl, Hiroshima, Nagasaki and Fukushima all released iodine 131. Indeed, as stated in the report by the US Institute of Medicine on Thyroid Screening Related to I-131 Exposure: 'A related memo estimated that an 11,000 to 212,000 excess cases of thyroid cancer were likely caused by the I-131.'[16] See also Chapter 6	If at risk of exposure, take higher doses of Lugol's iodine 15% (say 4 drops) twice daily (total daily dose 120 mg) to prevent the radioactive version being retained in the body

	X rays of the chest. Dental X rays may irradiate and damage the thyroid	Before any such investigation always inquire as to the possible gain. Always ask if this investigation will change management. So much medical investigation is mindless
	Medical imaging such as CT scanning uses very high doses of X rays	Ditto
	Medical imaging with radioactive isotopes	Ditto
	Medical imaging with gadolinium	Ditto
Amiodarone	This drug works to dispel cardiac dysrhythmias because it contains iodine. However, this is unnatural toxic iodine which eventually destroys the thyroid gland	
Lithium	Used to treat mania, but is toxic to the thyroid	Groundhog regimes work well to prevent mania[17]
Volatile organic compounds	Pesticides (including glyphosate aka 'Round up'), phthalates, organochlorine and formaldehyde all inhibit thyroid biochemistry	Do your best to avoid Detox – see below
Soya and cruciferous vegetables	This is not a problem so long as you have adequate iodine intake[18]	With a PK diet and all the above in place I would have no concerns with these foods. Again, Lugol's iodine 15% 3 drops daily – see Chapter 13

⁵Footnote: The Nevada Nuclear Bomb tests numbered in excess of 100 and took place mainly in the 1950s; these things often take decades before the truth comes out. As another example, there can be little doubt that the making of *The Conqueror* in St. George, Utah, resulted in several production members, including Susan Hayward, John Wayne, Agnes Moorehead, Pedro Armendáriz (who committed suicide after a diagnosis of cancer), and director Dick Powell all succumbing to cancer and cancer-related illnesses. As ascertained by *People* magazine in 1980, out of a cast and crew totalling 220 people, 91 of them developed some form of cancer, and 46 had died of the disease by that date. St. George, Utah, received the brunt of the fallout from above-ground nuclear testing at Nevada Test Site. Winds routinely carried the fallout of these tests directly through St. George and southern Utah.

Table 9.3: Traumatic or pathological injury to the thyroid (also see Chapter 6)

What	Why
Acute blood loss – for example, major obstetric haemorrhage	Drops the blood pressure and infarcts the pituitary gland (starves it of blood supply) so it underperforms for life. This results in secondary hypothyroidism. The adrenals may be similarly affected. When this is an obstetric bleed, it is called Sheehan's syndrome
Head injury	If the base of the skull has suffered fracture, then the blood supply to the pituitary may be impaired
Whiplash injury	I am not sure of the 'why' but there are several possible mechanisms

Tests of toxicity

Tests for toxic or heavy metals

As explained in Table 9.1, these are toxic because they are directly poisonous and/or they are immuno-toxic.

Measuring toxic metals in urine, blood or hair is unreliable because heavy metals are very poorly excreted and bio-concentrate in organs such as the heart, brain, bone marrow and kidneys. Consequently, they are not available to be measured. The answer is to use a chelating agent such as DMSA (captomer); this is well absorbed from the gut, grabs toxic and friendly minerals alike, and pulls them out through the urine. It is excellent for diagnosing toxicity of heavy metals such as mercury, lead, arsenic, aluminium, cadmium, nickel and probably others.[19] DMSA can be used to pull these metals out of the body through the urine. Expect also to see high readings of friendly minerals such as selenium, zinc, copper, manganese and chromium. If levels are not high, then that may point to a deficiency.

Immuno-toxicity of metals can be measured with MELISA testing (see https://melisa.org/).

Toxicity and immuno-toxicity go hand in hand. This makes perfect immunological sense and is an extension of normal immunity. If one has been poisoned by a metal or a virus, one becomes sensitised to this with, in the case of a virus, immunity and in the case of a metal, immuno-toxicity. The immune system has learned that these are baddies, remembers and swings into action with future exposures. The problem with metals is that, unlike viruses, they cannot be destroyed by inflammation. It is the persistent inflammation against an indestructible poisonous metal that drives pathology.

Tests for volatile organic compounds (VOCs) and pesticides

For this type of toxicity I recommend urine sampling here: www.greatplainslaboratory. com/gpl-tox. However, this is an expensive test. The bottom line is that we all carry a body burden of VOCs, and we should all do one heating regime a week to keep this as low as is possible. If you suspect you are poisoned, do these regimes as often as is possible (see Appendix F).

Tests for mycotoxins

If you suspect fungal infection or toxicity, I recommend urine sampling here: www. greatplainslaboratory.com/gplmycotox

How to reduce your toxic load

To deal with the toxic loads of metals, VOCs and/or mycotoxins you may be carrying, see Appendix F. This is repeated from our book *Ecological Medicine* – another mine of useful information. (I would say that wouldn't I?!#)

#**Historical note:** Marilyn Davies (1944 – 2014), known as Mandy Rice-Davies, was a model and showgirl and is best known for her association with Christine Keeler and her role in the so-called 'Profumo Affair'. Summarising and missing out some juicy details, in order to get to the point:
- John Profumo was the Secretary of State for War in Harold Macmillan's Conservative government and he had an extramarital affair with 19-year-old model Christine Keeler.
- As a result of revelations surrounding this affair, Stephen Ward, a friend of Keeler, was found guilty of living off immoral earnings and during the cross-examination at this trial, Rice-Davies made a remark, for which she is now famed. When James Burge, the defence counsel, stated that Lord Astor (also implicated) denied having an affair or even having met her, she dismissed this with, 'Well he would, wouldn't he?'

We have followed in the fine tradition of misquoting this quote by inserting a 'say'! There is a final twist to this quote – if one cannot be bothered to say the whole thing, then one merely says 'MRDA', meaning 'Mandy Rice-Davies applies'. What an incredible way to be remembered!

Can autoimmunity be reversed and switched off?

Probably autoimmunity can be reversed. Life is not a battle but a war – a war we know we are going to lose, but a war well worth fighting with all the tools of the trade detailed in this book and others. There is no single tool to switch off autoimmunity. You just have to put in place as many interventions as you possibly can and hope that your clever immune system will work it out and stop misbehaving.

Having said that, there are techniques to retrain the immune system – homeopathy, micro-immunotherapy and possibly meditation (an inflamed brain makes for an inflamed immune system). These are beyond the scope of this book, but what I do know is that the chances of success with these tools will be greatly enhanced by the Groundhog interventions alluded to throughout this book and detailed in the Appendices. Just do it!

Chapter 10

The hypothyroid child:
'Cretins', low IQ, failure to thrive
and Down's syndrome

The business of creating new life, developing babies in the womb and growing on to adulthood is hugely demanding of energy and raw materials. If the supply of energy or raw materials is impeded in any way, at any time, that child may not develop to its full potential – it will fail to thrive. Furthermore, any such failure is irreversible. So, for example we know that dyslexia is associated with zinc deficiency, but correcting such, once diagnosed, does not reverse the dyslexia. There is a critical window of time when the brain needs zinc to make the right connections and if this opportunity is missed then that loss is permanent.[1]

Nowhere is this truer than with hypothyroidism. So important is this that all babies are screened soon after birth with a heel prick test, the Guthrie test,* which includes a TSH score to test for hypothyroidism.

*__Historical note:__ The Guthrie test is named after Robert Guthrie MD PhD (1916 – 1995), an American microbiologist. This is another classic case of 'Follow the money' or '*cui bone*'[†] ('to whom is it a benefit?'), as the Romans said. Guthrie was told commercial production was the best and most efficient way to make the 400,000 test kits needed for his initial two-year study. He approached Ames Company, and Ames said it would only manufacture the kits if a patent was issued. Guthrie complied and filed a patent application in 1962, signing an exclusive licensing agreement with Miles, under which he would receive no royalties and 5% of the proceeds would be divided among the National Association for Retarded Children Research Fund, the Association for Aid of Crippled Children, and the University of Buffalo Foundation. But Miles couldn't produce the kits fast enough, and so Guthrie produced his own kits for 500 tests at a cost of $6 each. In 1963, Guthrie found out that Ames planned to charge $262 for the same kit. Guthrie was appalled, but Ames wouldn't lower their price. Eventually, after much legal wrangling, Guthrie won, and his trial was funded by US federal sources. Subsequently this led to the US Bayh–Dole Act which allows universities and small businesses to retain ownership of inventions developed with federal funding. But this just goes to show that it is money that drives Big Pharma and not care or compassion for the patient. Speaking of which, back to care and compassion....

Whilst in the womb, the baby's initial development is dependent on maternal thyroid hormones. These manifest from the very start of foetal life. The foetal thyroid begins concentrating iodine at 10-12 weeks of gestation and is under the control of foetal pituitary thyroid-stimulating hormone (TSH) by about 20 weeks of gestation, as described in the 2012 study by Angela M Leung.[2]

We know that the IQ of a child is inversely proportional to the mother's TSH (see Chapter 5, page 51). A low TSH gives us a healthy clever baby, a high TSH risks a 'cretin' – a baby severely physically and mentally disabled. Indeed, this is one of the reasons why obstetricians like the maternal TSH to be below 1.5. So do I! Indeed, as a general rule I like to see a TSH below 1.5 in all my patients. Why do some endocrinologists allow a TSH to run up to 5.0 in young women before treating them, when they may become pregnant next day… and thereby risk the life-long health of that baby?

The need for thyroid hormones increases perhaps by as much as 50% in pregnancy to cope with the additional demands of the developing baby – again, see Angela M Leung's study as above.[2] Any woman contemplating pregnancy should be checked for hypothyroidism. At the first sign of pregnancy, she should be re-checked, and this should be repeated during the second and third trimesters and again post-partum, when the need for thyroid hormones returns to normal. There is much detail about the management of pre-conception, pregnancy and more in our book *Green Mother*. Note in particular co-author Michelle's experience with carpal tunnel syndrome in pregnancy that was a warning sign of hypothyroidism – swelling related to low thyroid pressed on the carpal tunnel and told her she needed to supplement with thyroid glandular.

†**Linguistic note:** The expression '*cui bono*' is a 'double dative' construction – according to *Allen and Greenough's Latin Grammar for Schools and Colleges* (1893) only a few nouns are used in this construction which appears to be 'governed by custom, not by any principle'. This then is a gift to school girls and boys everywhere – anything goes! More formerly, the dative normally indicates an object or recipient, and the better-known example of a double dative, which normally has a 'dative of purpose', and a 'dative of reference' is with reference to Caesar in the Gallic Wars: '*suis saluti fuit*' – 'He was the salvation of his men',where the dative of the noun *salus, saluti* ('salvation'), expresses purpose and the dative of reference are his men being affected by this salvation. At this point,one simply has to link this clip from Monty Python's the *Life of Brian* – 'Romans Go Home' – where the incorrect use of the dative case causes the Roman Centurion to draw his sword! www.youtube.com/watch?v=IIAdHEwiAy8

Down's syndrome and hypothyroidism

So many doctors are happy to attribute all the features of Down's to genetics and thereby ignore interventions to allow these lovely, loving and gentle people to live to their full potential. Dr Henry Turkel showed how many of the lesions that flowed from having a third copy of chromosome 21 could be ameliorated by an ecological approach. Essentially, he applied Groundhog regimes in which the use of thyroid hormones was crucial. Down's syndrome shares many of the features of hypothyroidism and, indeed, hypothyroidism is common in Down's. I suspect it may be very common if not universal. Since thyroid hormones are so essential for the developing brain and body, the sooner this diagnosis is made, the better.

If you have a child with Down's, you will be very unlikely to find a doctor to help you. Read the work of Dr Turkel and just do it. As an introduction, see his 'Medical Amelioration of Down's Syndrome Incorporating the Orthomolecular Approach', published in 1975 and freely available online.[3]

Chapter 11

The hypothyroid female:
Puberty and PMT, infertility,
pregnancy, menopause

Hypothyroidism is more common in females than males and this has much to do with female sex hormones. To quote Birte Nygaard in *BMJ Clinical Evidence*, 'Hypothyroidism is six times more common in women, affecting up to 40/10,000 each year (compared with 6/10,000 men).'[1] Why so?

There is only one evolutionary reason why we exist and that is for the purpose of procreation. Interested readers may like to read the 2013 article by Andrew Rifkin, 'Is the meaning of life to make babies' in *Scientific American*,[2] which looks at many reasons for existence, but does conclude that, from the evolutionary point of view, the answer is a resounding 'yes!'.

For the purposes of such, the whole evolutionary drive is diverted to the advantage of the baby and if Mother's survival is compromised in that process, then so be it. Having babies is a very dangerous business for women and many die as a result of complications of impregnation (sexually transmitted disease), pregnancy, childbirth and post-partum problems (blood loss, puerperal fever, postnatal depression).

Even taking a crude measure of maternal deaths relating to pregnancy and childbirth only, and only looking at the six-month post-partum period, one woman dies every two minutes, with a further 20-30 suffering significant injury, infection or disability every two minutes also.[3] Of course, a healthy mother is desirable, but not essential, for her baby's survival. Be in no doubt, that evolutionary imperative means baby comes first.

Procreation is hugely demanding of energy and raw materials. Female fertility comes with the production of female sex hormones and primitive woman was rarely fertile. She rarely experienced a menstrual bleed because either she was too young, pregnant, breast-feeding, menopausal or simply starving. On the rare occasion when none of these applied, there would be a flood of sex hormones to switch on all those attributes to attract a male and allow that mental state of madness which permits that highly dangerous activity of sexual intercourse! It takes energy to be attractive to others – energy to be sociable, energy to be physically active and energy to be mentally fascinating. These are powerful signals to a sexual partner and clearly indicate that abundance of energy essential for the rearing of children. Our book, *Green Mother*, contains much more detail.

I always used to wonder why my mother said, 'Child-rearing is a young woman's game'. I know now – it is all about energy! With such an understanding of evolutionary imperatives and mechanisms of action we can see why it is that female sex hormones, natural or synthetic, endogenous (produced by the body) or exogenous (from the Pill and HRT) are so dangerous: they are correlated with energy, in that they will not be produced when energy is in short supply.

Female sex hormones and immune tolerance

From an immunological perspective, the baby is a tissue transplant. Up to half its genetics are foreign. Logically Mother's immune system should simply reject the growing foetus, and indeed, this is a recognised cause of miscarriage. Female sex hormones are immuno-suppressive, and this induces immune tolerance to suppress this immunological rejection. However, if you disturb immune tolerance, you increase the risk of autoimmunity, and hypothyroidism is one of the commonest autoimmune conditions. Moulton (2018) discussed this relationship, noting that: 'The female predilection of autoimmune diseases ranging from 3:1 for MS to 15:1 for autoimmune thyroiditis clearly implicates the female gender and sex hormones in autoimmunity.'[4]

Female sex hormones and immunosuppression

The Pill blunts the immune response to all infections – yeast and fungi (such as candida), viruses and bacteria. Viruses may infect the thyroid gland directly and/or switch on autoimmunity (see Chapter 7 and Moulton's paper[4]).

Female sex hormones and micronutrient deficiencies

Female sex hormones prioritise expenditure of energy and micro-nutrients to the business of procreation. Mother 'pays' for this with her own health.

Female sex hormones and energy

Sex hormones that arise naturally from good health carefully match energy availability to demands. They will not be produced when energy is in short supply. This is why exogenous sex hormones such as the Pill, HRT and 'natural, bio-identical' hormone creams are so dangerous. They give the body the false impression that it has energy to spend. That may result in fun in the short term but, as I know, energy availability, or rather lack of it, drives pathology. Without the energy for healing and repair we descend into degenerative conditions such as dementia, heart disease and cancer. The Pill and HRT are risk factors for all these conditions.

Recognising these dangers, the 'Citizens' Petition on Hormonal Contraceptives June 2019' was filed with the FDA (the USA's Food and Drug Administration) requesting more transparency and patient warnings regarding potential side effects for different forms of hormonal contraceptives, including breast cancer, cervical cancer, inflammatory bowel disease, systemic lupus erythematosus (SLE), depression and suicide, venous thrombosis and cardiovascular events, multiple sclerosis (MS) and bone fracture. This document is 98 pages long and references dozens of studies so is well worth the read if you want to know more.[5]

See also the 2019 open-acess paper by the Collaborative Group on Hormonal Factors in Breast Cancer which concluded that: 'In western countries there have been about 20 million breast cancers diagnosed since 1990, of which about 1 million would have been caused by MHT use.'[6]

The false energy of sex hormones masks the true energy deficit of hypothyroidism and this manifests at key periods in a woman's life, including at puberty and menopause.

Puberty

Puberty marks the moment when children become fertile. The age of puberty is falling.

In 1860, the average age of the onset of puberty in girls was 16.6 years. In 1920, it was 14.6; in 1950, 13.1; in 1980, 12.5; and in 2010, it had dropped to 10.5. Similar sets of figures have been reported for boys, albeit with a delay of around a year.[7] Why so?

There are at least two reasons: pollution (oestrogen mimics) and Western diets. Age of puberty is largely determined by food availability—for obvious evolutionary reasons. In the West, we now live in a state of calorie abundance and obesity but nutritional inadequacy. It is now considered normal to see pubertal changes in girls as young as 7, boys as young as 8. This is not desirable for many reasons beyond the scope of this chapter. However, these early surges of hormones may well mask hypothyroidism in children.

If puberty is delayed from the 'new normal', the anxiety which arises from such may drive the GP to prescribe the Pill. This is, however, very poor medicine. The Pill drives an artificial puberty which the body in question is simply not ready for. Pituitary hormone production is switched off and the girl may be rendered infertile for life.

The commonest cause of delayed puberty in Westerners today is hypothyroidism.

Periods and PMT

As detailed above, seeing a period is an evolutionary anomaly. However, a regular, light, painless menstrual bleed, free from PMT is an excellent sign of good nutrition, good thyroid function and so fertility – not my words but those of Margaret and Arthur Wynn who devoted their lives to the study of women's health and nutrition, with diet, iodine sufficiency and hypothyroidism being big players. As they noted in a 1991 publication, the menstrual cycle signs of toxicity correlate with not only markers of nutritional adequacy, but also with hormone-driven disease such as diabetes and hypothyroidism.[8] The treatment of these problems is to put in place Groundhog Basic (see Appendix D), and then sort the thyroid.

Infertility

It is estimated that one in seven UK couples has difficulty conceiving (approximately 3.5 million people).[9] Infertility arises for many reasons (see our book *Green Mother*), but a common reason is poor energy delivery mechanisms (Nature is telling you that you do not have the resources for healthy offspring). I have seen many infertile couples who can be easily and effectively treated with Groundhog Basic (Appendix D), eliminating sexually transmitted diseases and sorting out the thyroid.

Pregnancy and post-partum depression

The requirement for thyroid hormones increases by 50% during pregnancy, according to Singh and Sandhu (2022): 'During pregnancy, thyroid hormone production increases by around 50% along with a similar increase in total daily iodine requirements.'[10]

This means that the borderline hypothyroid woman may tip into overt hypothyroidism during pregnancy. This has dire effects for the growing baby – the worse the hypothyroidism, the lower the IQ of the baby (see Chapters 5 and 10). Hypothyroidism also has dire effects on Mother, with the risk of miscarriage, pre-eclampsia (dangerously high blood pressure), anaemia, placenta praevia and postpartum haemorrhage all being increased.

All women should have thyroid checks before pregnancy, during pregnancy and when there is any hint of post-partum depression. Depression may well be symptomatic of poor energy delivery mechanisms and this horrible condition may respond dramatically to Groundhog Basic and sorting the thyroid.

Menopause

So many symptoms, especially those of poor energy delivery (see Chapter 1) are falsely attributed to the menopause. The knee-jerk reaction of many therapists is to prescribe female sex hormones, but this is dangerous medicine, with all the complications of female sex hormones as detailed above. The Million Women HRT Study had to be abandoned at 18 months because of the excess cancers in the hormone-taking group. Life expectancy was shortened. As the researchers have reported on the Nuffield Department of Population Health website:

> *After crunching through all the data, Beral and her team – notably statistician Professor Gillian Reeves – found that women who were currently using HRT were at an increased risk of breast cancer. This risk was significantly larger for women taking combined HRT containing the hormones oestrogen and progestogen, compared to oestrogen-only pills.*

Since then, the Million Women Study has revealed that HRT can also increase the risk of ovarian cancer, while oestrogen-only HRT increases the risk of endometrial (womb) cancer. Taken together, breast, ovarian and womb cancer add up to 40 per cent of all female cancers in the UK, affecting many tens of thousands of women. Overall, over a five-year period, for every thousand women not taking HRT, around 19 of them will develop one of these diseases. For 1000 women taking oestrogen-only HRT this goes up to 26, and up to 34 cancers for every 1000 women taking combined HRT.[11]

Improving energy delivery mechanisms, with special attention to the thyroid and adrenals, cures many symptoms attributed to the menopause. The most difficult symptom is the hot flushes. We know these are directly due to lack of female sex hormones because they are reliably abolished with the prescription of such. Not an option! But this gives us clues to the mechanisms. The menopause arises because women run out of their finite supply of eggs. Unfortunately, the pituitary gland does not know this, the evolutionary imperative to procreate persists and the pituitary pours out higher and higher levels of follicle stimulating hormone (FSH) and luteinising hormone (LH) to kick the ovaries into life for one last pregnancy. These hormones are released in pulses and a high pulse of such has a bradykinin-mimicking action (bradykinin is a peptide that promotes inflammation) to cause profound vasodilatation with flushing – most uncomfortable.

Correcting thyroid and adrenal function mitigates but does not abolish the hot flush. The only happy thought is that hot flushes must be symptomatic of good energy delivery mechanisms and so those suffering from them should live longer!

Light relief: In celebration of femaleness, by Craig

So far, it looks like there are many disadvantages to being a woman. We all know this is untrue and so it falls upon me [Craig] to redress the balance a little before the reader moves on. Quoting men's thoughts about women, and celebrating the female, sometimes in a humorous way, seems like a good way to discharge this responsibility. Robert Heinlein (1907 – 1988, American science fiction writer), perceptive as always, remarked that women and cats will always do as they want, and that men and dogs should get used to it! Others have put it equally well:

To call woman the weaker sex is a libel; it is man's injustice to woman. If by strength is meant brute strength, then, indeed, is woman less brute than man. If by strength is meant moral power, then woman is immeasurably man's superior. Has she not greater intuition, is she not more self-sacrificing, has she not greater powers of endurance, has she not greater courage? Without her, man could not be. If nonviolence is the law of our being, the future is with woman. Who can make a more effective appeal to the heart than woman?
To the Women of India (Young India, 4 October 1930)
Mahatma Gandhi, 1869 – 1948 (assassinated), Indian lawyer and political ethicist

And one of my favourite quotes of all time:

What would men be without women? Scarce, sir... mighty scarce.
Mark Twain, 1835 – 1910, American writer, humourist, entrepreneur, publisher, and lecturer

And to end, we have Aesop:

Fire, woman and sea, the mighty three.
Πυρ, γυνή και θάλασσα, δυνατά τρία
Aesop, 620 – 560 BC, Ancient Greek fabulist

Chapter 12

Thyrotoxicosis:
Autoimmunity, nodules and cancer

Thankfully the conditions I've reserved for this Chapter are rare. You will need medical input from an endocrinologist to deal with any of them, but much more can be done besides and you will almost certainly need to take charge of long-term follow up of any medical or surgical treatment you have.

Thyrotoxicosis

This is the clinical picture (combination of symptoms and signs) that emerges when there is a pathological outpouring of thyroid hormones. The accelerator pedal of your mitochondrial engine is flat to the boards and in the short term you appear to have limitless energy. It is like being on amphetamine and some initially love that feeling. However, it is very damaging in the longer term. As ever, normalising thyroid function is the key.

Symptoms include:
- uncontrolled and increased energy delivery, causing insomnia
- feeling too hot
- heightened physical and mental powers
- often heightened mood, sometimes with psychiatric manifestations of mania or psychosis
- weight loss: this outpouring of energy burns precious fat resources
- heart symptoms: the heart beats more powerfully and faster, with tachycardia, perhaps dysrhythmias (palpitations) and high blood pressure, sweating and muscle weakness.

Signs (what examination and testing pick up) include:

- fast pulse
- higher body temperatures
- high blood pressure
- tremor
- sweaty and shaky hands
- anxiety: some sufferers feel intensely anxious
- bulging eyes or 'exophthalmos' (so you can see the white of the eye all around the iris). The mechanism of this is probably autoimmune.

It is important to recognise that Graves' disease (autoimmune hyperthyroid), or thyrotoxicosis from another cause (see below), is a clinical picture confirmed by blood tests. It is not – or should not be – diagnosed from blood tests alone. Sadly, many doctors do this: they recognise thyrotoxicosis on the basis of a suppressed TSH level and patients end up being under-treated – this often occurs after thyrotoxicosis has been over-treated because thyroid levels have not been checked and patients left on high doses of carbimazole too long.

Having established the clinical picture we then have to look for the cause, which gives us a proper diagnosis.

Causes of thyrotoxicosis

1. An autoimmune response. Thyrotropin (TSH) receptor antibody (TRAb) testing is considered accurate for the diagnosis of Graves' disease (GD)* and this test is

---

Historical note: Graves' disease is named after Robert James Graves FRCS (1796 – 1853), an eminent Irish surgeon. Robert Graves died of liver disease at his country residence, 20 March 1853, one week before his 57th birthday, far too young. He led a varied life. For example, during a gale in the Mediterranean, the ship on which he was a passenger sprang a leak and, worse still, the pumps failed. The crew were about to abandon ship. Instead, Graves holed the one lifeboat with an axe, and shouted, 'Let us all be drowned together, it is a pity to part good company'. He then repaired the pumps with leather from his own shoes and saved the ship and all its company and passengers.[9] He is also the uncredited inventor of the second hand on wristwatches and, following his death, a Dublin watchmaking company began selling watches with second hands, Graves having not patented his idea.[10] These kinds of polymath seem few and far between these days. A few years ago, Sarah passed on to me her copy of the book *The Last Man who Knew Everything*, a biography of the British polymath Thomas Young, detailing his achievements in areas such as physics (e.g. Young's modulus), mathematics, physiology, medicine (e.g. Young's rule), linguistics and Egyptology. And to top it all, this amazing individual was modest, understated and generous to others with his genius. Well worth a read. Craig.

essential. The point here is that if negative then one must look for other causes such as 2 and 3 below.

2. A 'hot nodule'. This is an adenoma – a lump – in the thyroid gland which, for reasons unknown, produces excessive thyroid hormones uncontrollably. It can be diagnosed by radioactive iodine scan to show increased uptake of iodine.

3. Thyroid cancer. Thankfully rare, accounting for just 1% of all new cancer cases in 2016-2018 in the UK[1] but not to be overlooked. It is diagnosed by biopsy of the nodule. It needs removing surgically. In the long term, sufficient thyroid replacement therapy should be given to keep the TSH level low – certainly below 0.5 mIU/l. Why? Because TSH is a growth promoter. Thyroid cancer is much more common in women than men (2.9 times according to Rahbari et al[2]) because of the growth-promoting effects of female sex hormones.

Treatment of thyrotoxicosis

Thyrotoxicosis may be a medical emergency and in the very short term the effects of thyroid hormones must and can be blocked by beta-blocking drugs. There is then a rather poor choice for the patient between carbimazole, surgery or radiation. I would always advocate the first (if the individual can tolerate it[†]).

- **Carbimazole:** This is given in high doses initially – 15-40 mg daily – then titrated down over the ensuing weeks. Time for titration varies depending on patient response but the Cochrane Review of 26 studies concluded that 12 months was superior to six months, but that there was no benefit in extending treatment beyond 18 months.[3] At the same time, put in place interventions that tackle autoimmunity (PK diet, vitamin D 10,000 iu daily and avoid vaccination, see Chapter 9). This

---

[†]**Explanatory note:** Carbimazole is a 'pro-drug'; after absorption it is converted to the active form, methimazole. Methimazole prevents thyroid peroxidase enzyme from iodinating and coupling the tyrosine residues on thyroglobulin, hence reducing the production of the thyroid hormones T3 and T4. Please check that you are a good candidate for using it:

- Have you ever had an allergic reaction to it in the past? Signs of a previous allergic reaction are a sudden rash, swelling or difficulty breathing.
- Have you ever had severe pancreatic issues after taking carbimazole in the past? If acute pancreatitis occurs during treatment, immediately and permanently stop the drug. Re-exposure to carbimazole may result in life-threatening acute pancreatitis with a decreased time to onset
- Are you pregnant or trying for a baby? Carbimazole is associated with an increased risk of congenital malformations, especially when administered in the first trimester of pregnancy and at high doses.

may reduce the antibody titre but will certainly reduce your risk of developing other autoimmune diseases.

- **Surgery:** This is never without potential for complications. The parathyroid glands reside within the thyroid and may be damaged by surgery. Calcium levels must be monitored post-operatively, possibly for life.
- **Radioactive iodine:** This is reserved for those who cannot tolerate or are not fit for carbimazole or surgery. It involves a high dose of radiation and so you risk triggering a cancer elsewhere in the body. If there were no option, I would allow a couple of days for the treatment to work, then use high-dose iodine as per Chapter 13 (page 105) to dislodge any remaining radioactive iodine. (Incidentally, in the event of a nuclear accident that releases radioactive iodine, iodine 50 mg daily prevents the radioactive stuff getting stuck in the body to cause cancer.)

Treatment follow-up

This is where the endocrinologists seem to lose interest. With any of the above treatments, it is all too easy to overshoot and end up underactive (see Chapter 6). Indeed, surgeons and radiotherapists will always err on the side of over-treatment because it is relatively easy to correct the underactive thyroid, and no one wants a second dose of surgery or radiotherapy. What this means is that you must monitor your thyroid symptoms and signs very closely (see Chapter 1) and back this up with blood tests, initially every two weeks, then adjust the frequency as you get a feel for the rate of progress. If there is any doubt at any stage, retest.

If the thyrotoxicosis is due to autoimmunity, then this increases the risk of other autoimmune conditions.[4] The risk factors for all are vaccinations (avoid), vitamin D deficiency (we all need 10,000 iu daily), dairy protein and gluten (yes – it is that PK diet again!) – see Chapters 1, 2 and 6.

Thyroid cancer

Thyroid cancer is becoming more common, probably because iodine deficiency is on the increase and because the diagnosis of hypothyroidism is being missed or undertreated. In both these cases, the TSH is raised. TSH is a growth promoter as discussed before.

Obviously, any tumour needs excising. After that, the key is to use thyroid hormones to keep the TSH well suppressed, and this prevents recurrence. In parallel you also need to do Groundhog Chronic (see Appendix D). Cancer cells can only survive on sugar and carbs and hence the PK diet is the starting point. Then take vitamin C to bowel tolerance as this kills cancer cells.[5, 6, 7, 8]

What about iodine? This too has anticancer properties – see Chapter 13. Read on!

Chapter 13

Iodine

Iodine is a vital multitasking tool whose full potential has yet to be realised. Big Pharma's powerful propaganda machine has seen to that because iodine deficiency is a major driver of pathology. Pathology demands prescription medicines and thereby profits.

How safe is iodine

Iodine is very safe. During the first half of the 20th century, almost every US physician used Lugol's solution for iodine supplementation in his/her practice for both hypo- and hyperthyroidism and many other medical conditions. The minimum dose was 6.25 mg of elemental iodine with the recommended daily intake being 12.5 to 37.5 mg.[1]

In 1995, this was still the recommended dose in the 19th edition of *Remington's Science and Practice of Pharmacy*.[2] Nobel Laureate Albert Szent-Gyorgyi* commented: 'When I was a medical student, iodine in the form of KI was the universal medicine. Nobody knew what it did, but it did something and did something good. We students used to sum up the situation in this little rhyme: 'If you do not know where, what and why, prescribe ye then K and I.'[3]

*Historical note:** Albert Szent-Gyorgyi, 1893 –1986, was a Hungarian biochemist who won the Nobel Prize in Physiology or Medicine in 1937. He is credited with first isolating vitamin C and discovering the components and reactions of the citric acid cycle.

Iodine sufficiency

Iodine insufficiency is pandemic. Iodine deficiency is common. It is the former that is most important – that dose of iodine for optimal health. Even today the normal daily requirement of the body for iodine has not been determined. The body cannot store iodine, so it takes what is necessary from the diet and excretes the rest. So where do we need iodine and why?

Table 13.1: How the body uses iodine

Organ	Notes	References
Thyroid	Thyroxin, T4 so named as it contains four iodine atoms. Tri-iodothyronine, T3, so named as it contains three iodine atoms	See Chapter 1
Heart	Dr B West states, 'Most of the stubborn cases of cardiac arrhythmias and atrial fibrillation that we were unable to completely correct with our cardiac protocols have now been resolved with adequate supplies of iodine added.' The commonest dysrhythmia is ventricular ectopics. In addition to iodine 50 mg at night, also use magnesium 300 mg and vitamin D 10,000 iu per day and cut out caffeine and chocolate	Iodine Research – The Resource Network of the Iodine Movement http://iodineresearch.com/heart.html
	The therapeutic effect of the antidysrhythmic drug amiodarone may result because it is delivering high doses of iodine (albeit in a toxic form)	
Immune system – cancer	Japanese women have the lowest rates of breast cancer in the world. A 2003 report published in the journal *Breast Cancer Research* postulated that this could be a direct result of eating iodine- and selenium-rich seaweed, which is a staple in the Japanese diet. Iodine is an antioxidant and anti-proliferative and so protective against	Smyth (2003)[4] Aceves et al (2013)[5]

Auto-immunity	'Iodine deficiency, not excess, is the cause of autoimmune thyroid disease'	BMJ Rapid Response by Peter Lewis, General Practitioner with special interest in Integrative Medicine to Niranjan et al (2016) 'Should we treat subclinical hypothyroidism in obese children?' with eight references[6, 7]
Breast tissue	Fibrocystic disease and breast pain can be reversed with iodine sufficiency	Ghent et al (1993)[8]
Fat	Without iodine, one cannot fat burn. The more fat carried, the more iodine is required	Abraham[9]
Brain	The most common and yet preventable cause of mental impairment is iodine deficiency	Redman et al (2016)[10]
	'Currently, ID [iodine deficiency] disorders are the single greatest contributor to preventable brain damage in fetuses and infants and arrested psycho-motor development in children'	Choudhry & Nasrullah (2018)[11]
Sleep	The toxic brain does not sleep. Iodine is a great detoxifier (see Chapter 9) Iodine is essential for quality sleep. Many report the return of dreaming with adequate iodine	
Skin	...and without it the skin cannot sweat	Chelson (2017)[12]
Energy delivery mechanisms	Many report better energy and wellbeing with iodine sufficiency. Mitochondria need iodine to work and as an antioxidant	Dillon & Hoch (1967): 'The total iodine content of liver mitochondria obtained from hypothyroid rats was about 20% of that mitochondria from normal rats'[13]
Striated muscle	Muscle pain may be a symptom of iodine insufficiency	
Bone	The lower the iodine the greater the risk of osteoarthritis and osteoporosis	Arslanca et al (2018)[14]

Table 13.1 (cont'd)

Organ	Notes	References
Sex hormones	There are three oestrogens, the mother oestrone E1 which may convert into one of two offspring – namely, oestradiol E2 (a pre-carcinogen) or oestriol E3 (cancer protective). Iodine directs E1 to the friendly E3 and this is protective against hormone sensitive cancers	Deville (2015)[15]
Temp-erature control	The lower the urinary iodine the greater the frequency and severity of hot flushes in menopausal women	Korkmaz et al (2015)[16]

How much iodine do we need for sufficiency?

A normal thyroid gland contains 50 mg of iodine, fat in the body and breast tissue contain 700 mg, and striated muscle contains 650 mg. Altogether 20% of body iodine (about 400 mg) is present in the skin. Iodine sufficiency means we need a total body load of at least 1.5 possibly 2 grams – that is, 2000 mg or 2,000,000 mcg.[17]

The risible Recommended Daily Amount is 150 mcg in the UK[18] (and even lower at 140 in the US[19]) which means it would take 13,333 days to achieve iodine sufficiency... if no iodine was excreted. The fact is it is impossible to achieve sufficiency with such a miserly dose.

Iodine sufficiency is defined when 90% of an oral dose is excreted. This figure has been worked out clinically by Drs Abraham, Brownstein and Flechas. Most individuals in their study needed 37.5-50 mg of iodine daily for up to two years before achieving and maintaining sufficiency.[9] This makes much more sense – to achieve a body load of 2000 mg would need 40 days of 50 mg of iodine, assuming none was excreted... which of course it is! Like vitamin C, it is a wonderful multitasking tool, and it is only when it has achieved the jobs listed in Table 13.1 and satisfied our tissue requirements that we achieve a stable state of iodine sufficiency.

Above all, human existence requires stability, the permanence of things.
Georges Albert Maurice Victor Bataille (1897 – 9 July 1962), French philosopher
and intellectual

How to take iodine

Start low and build up slowly for two reasons:
1. To avoid the Wolff-Chaikoff effect (see below)
2. Because you may get detox reactions (as you clear our toxic metals and halides) and die-off reactions (as you clean up the upper fermenting gut) – see Appendix G.

Do not take iodine at the same time (i.e. 'exactly' the same time) as vitamin C. It is an oxidising agent (electron receiver) whilst vitamin C is a reducing agent (electron donor). They knock each other out. Vitamin C is best taken little and often through the day in water. So, take iodine last thing at night in a glass of water, at least one hour away from vitamin C. Build up to 50 mg at night. Big people need more than little people.

Table 13.2: How much iodine is in a drop of Lugol's? Lugol's is a combination of iodine and potassium iodide

Lugol's %	Iodine content in mg (free iodine)	Iodide content in mg (potassium iodide)	Total iodine available to the body in mg	Number of drops to deliver 50 mg
2%	1	1.5	2.5	20
3%	1.5	2.25	3.75	14
5%	2.5	3.75	6.25	8
7%	3.5	5.25	8.75	5-6
10%	5	7.5	12.5	4
12%	6	9	15	3-4
15%	7.5	11.25	18.75	3

The problems for which we need iodine the most

Iodine is used up in the business of getting rid of the upper fermenting gut and detoxing heavy metals and bromides.

Treating the upper fermenting gut

A Western carb-based diet almost invariably results in an upper fermenting gut (see Chapter 3). Iodine contact-kills all microbes at 10 parts per million (that is, 10 mg per litre of water).[20, 21] To confirm this, see the World Health Organization's report *Iodine as a drinking-water disinfectant* (2018) for many examples and Eggers (2019), in particular for Table 1 which confirms efficacy against bacteria, bacteria spores and enveloped and non-enveloped viruses.

Since this is the first port of call for ingested iodine, its first job is to sterilise the upper gut. This is greatly facilitated by a PK diet.

Excreting toxic metals

We all carry a load of toxic metals because we live in such a toxic world. We know iodine increases the excretion of lead, mercury, cadmium and aluminium.[9]

Excreting toxic fluoride and bromide

Fluorides and bromides are highly toxic. Both may cause hypothyroidism. The effect is worse where there is iodine deficiency, as the thyroid gland may make a biochemical error and pick up bromide or fluoride instead. Iodine sufficiency reverses this and we see excretion of these toxic halides in urine.[9]

Getting rid of the upper fermenting gut and detoxing heavy metals and bromides, together with restoring iodine for thyroid function, adrenal function, production of oxytocin and sex hormones, improving antioxidant status and improving mitochondrial function results in a feeling of wellbeing.

How do we know if iodine sufficiency has been achieved?

Iodine sufficiency is defined as being when all the pathologies detailed in Table 13.1, thanks to iodine supplementation done alongside Groundhog Chronic regimes, have been abolished. However, it is always good to have a test. As we know, 90% of an oral dose is excreted. Any less than this means it is going into body stores – that is, you are deficient.

Iodine sufficiency is assessed by an iodine loading test. The test consists of 50 mg iodine/iodide (see Table 13.2). Collect urine for 24 hours, measure the volume and send a sample to the relevant lab. If your body is healthily saturated with iodine (that is, iodine sufficient) then 90% of the ingested iodine will pass out in the 24-hour urine sample. This test is available at Regenerus Labs: https://regeneruslabs.com/products/urine-iodine-1

Experience tells us that it takes at least three months of 50 mg daily to achieve iodine sufficiency, so there is little point in doing the test if this level of iodine has not been consumed. It maybe self-evident from the symptom improvement that sufficiency has been achieved and renders testing unnecessary. The important point is that no-one has ever become iodine toxic on 50 mg of natural iodine – it is all too easily excreted![9]

Can iodine be toxic?

Iodine can only do good so long as you start low and go slow. This is important because without supplementation you will be deficient. So, in receipt of an acute large dose, the thyroid gland will give a metaphorical 'yippee' and go into over-production. This is called the Wolff-Chaikoff effect. It only lasts one or two weeks at which point normal function is restored. Some may feel thyrotoxic during this window of time.

Should iodine be used in hyperthyroidism or thyrotoxicosis?

Yes, iodine should be used with overactive thyroid because, as Table 13.1 shows, it is not just needed for the thyroid. It is present in all cells of the body and is in particular demand in breast tissue, the brain, immune system (concentrates in mucous membranes of the respiratory tract and gut for infection defence), skin and fat.

Should iodine be used in autoimmune disease?

Yes, iodine should be used in autoimmune disease for all the above reasons.

What about iodine allergy or toxicity?

Iodine allergy is not a problem with natural iodine such as Lugol's. It is only a problem with man-made synthetic versions, such as iodine-containing compounds for radio-imaging, radioactive iodine, or drugs containing iodine, such as amiodarone.

Many people are told that allergy to shell fish means they are allergic to iodine – nonsense!

Iodine as an antimicrobial

Iodine contact-kills all microbes at a concentration of 10 parts per million (often less). It is the only agent that is consistently active against gram positive and gram-negative bacteria, mycobacteria, spores, amoebic cysts, fungi, protozoa, yeasts, drug-resistant bacteria such as MRSA and viruses. In the doses below, it is non-toxic to the immune system cells responsible for healing and repair – indeed, studies show it enhances healing. This is why surgeons love it. Skin painted with iodine before incision does not get infected and heals perfectly.[22] There is much more detail in our book *The Infection Game: Life is an arms race*.

Furthermore, iodine is volatile and so it can get to areas that vitamin C cannot. Even if it cannot be applied directly to the infected area, it will penetrate flesh easily and is carried in the air to be inhaled. Infection is hit from within by vitamin C and from without by iodine. I use it in two ways to deal with infection and, indeed, Lugol's iodine, a salt pipe and coconut oil should be essential tools in your first aid box.

To treat all conditions of the mouth and airways

These conditions include: gingivitis (gum disease), pharyngitis, tonsillitis, rhinitis, sinusitis, laryngitis, bronchitis, chest infections and bronchiectasis.

Use a salt pipe to deliver the iodine. This is simply a plastic pot filled with sea salt that can be used as an inhaler. Drizzle Lugol's iodine 15% 2 drops into the mouthpiece to 'load' the salt pipe with iodine. Place the mouthpiece under your nose and sniff …then exhale through your mouth. If you can smell the iodine, you have received a therapeutic dose. Do five to 10 such sniffs. Perhaps use the Valsalva manoeuvre to blow the iodine vapour into the middle ear and sinuses – pinch your nose and blow into it so your ears pop (see http://goflightmedicine.com/clearing-ears/). Do this at least three times daily but as often as you can according to the severity of the infection. In the short term, expect to see more catarrh as your body sweeps out the dead microbes.

For a child who cannot manage a salt pipe, smear the nostrils and lips with a coconut oil/iodine mix. The volatile iodine will be inhaled. You will have to think of a good joke to explain the necessity for a yellow nose and mouth!

To treat all skin conditions and superficial pathology

This includes such problems as infected spots, chicken pox, cold sores, swollen lymph nodes, nail infections, ear infections, cradle cap, skin fungal infections (tinea, ringworm, acne, boils), scabs and bruises.

Take 100 ml of coconut oil and place the pot in a warm place so the oil just melts. Stir in 10 ml of Lugols 15% iodine to give you a 1.5% mix. Coconut oil is additionally beneficial as this is viricidal and is the fuel that powers the immune system, also further helping the healing and repair process.[23]

Just as with vitamin C, the key is in the dose. Iodine can only kill if present. You know it is present because you can see the yellow colour. You must apply it as often as necessary to keep the area stained yellow/orange/brown (but not so much as to 'pickle' the skin).

For lymph node swelling

Swollen lymph nodes are often called 'glands' but they are not, as one may see in acute tonsillitis, glandular fever and local skin infections. Ask the question 'why?' and assess if it is any of the following. If none of these, then blood tests will be needed and medical opinion (it could be a lymphoma or secondary cancer spread).

Parotitis (for example, mumps)

This refers to swelling of the parotid 'glands'. I saw one case of mumps disappear overnight with topical ad lib iodine oil. Yes, the iodine stain did make her look like some

---

†**Linguistic note:** Once again, we are aware that the reader may be in need of some light relief. One of the most frequent words in this book is 'Lugol's'. The leading 'L' is an example of a 'liquid consonant' – in phonetics, this is a consonant sound in which the tongue produces a partial closure in the mouth, and which results in a resonant, vowel-like consonant, such as English 'l' and 'r'. Say 'Lugol's' and note where your tongue is – it most likely will be touching your hard palate at the top of the inside of your mouth. The same happens with liquid, ironically.

kind of alien, but she felt so much better. I have yet to try this with a mumps orchitis – I can hardly wait for the opportunity!

Vaginal and perineal infections

Warm your iodine oil so it melts and steep tampons in it. Allow to cool so the oil solid-ifies. Use at least twice daily, possibly more often. This has the potential to contact-kill any vaginal infection and possibly viruses occupying the cervix.

Eye infections

These include blepharitis, conjunctivitis and iritis.

Do not put the iodine oil into the eye. Smear it over the eyelids and the iodine will evaporate and get into the eye.

Alternatively, use povidone-iodine which does not sting the eye. This does not work as well as Lugol's as the iodine is bound up so it does not penetrate as well.

Wounds, ulcers or broken skin

Any injuries of this sort must be kept still to allow the immune system to build new flesh. This is where pain is such a vital symptom because it ensures such. The wound should be fully debrided, comfortably dressed in non-sticky gauze and a bandage. Keep this dressing undisturbed for at least a week, but drizzle pure Lugol's onto the outside of the dressing. The volatile iodine will keep the wound infection free so it can heal without disturbing the rebuilding process. I have to say this works very well with dogs and horses too.

Warts and veruccas

Put a spot of pure Lugol's iodine directly onto the lesion. Keep it stained brown. It will kill the virus, but you must keep applying iodine for several weeks until the skin has grown out the lesion.

Insect bites

I carry Lugol's iodine 15% all the time. It happens that I am anaphylactic to wasp stings having suffered such as a child. Whilst gardening in Spring 2020 I was stung on the arm. Within seconds a red swelling came up and as I set off for the antihistamines and adrenalin I thought 'iodine!' I painted the lump yellow with neat Lugol's and within minutes the swelling, redness and itch had completely abated.

I also get severe itchy reactions to horse fly and midge bites. Lugol's has the same dramatic effect. My experience has been paralleled by others.

Many diseases are transmitted by insect bites. This is further reason to apply Lugol's – one may nip Lyme disease in the bud!

Is thyroid replacement therapy needed for life? The theory

People invariably ask me if thyroid replacement therapy is for life. Hitherto I have said yes, but now I am not so sure.

From an evolutionary perspective, there must have come a moment, or series of moments, when those animals with the most energy prevailed. Energy was not limitless, and so control mechanisms had to evolve. Perhaps iodine was the original accelerator pedal? This would make sense because highly nutritious diets would have been paralleled by high iodine content. Primitive life‡ probably evolved in water where iodine would have been super-abundant. The more food consumed, the more iodine and the greater the energy levels available for physical and mental activity.

One can imagine a situation where the intelligent body noticed this parallel and adapted accordingly. However, as primitive life moved onto land, so the iodine content of the diet fell. Perhaps these independent beasts adapted by holding iodine in a carrier protein that increased its power to stimulate energy generation. Thus, were thyroid hormones spawned.

Iodine, of course, is the atom within thyroid hormones that renders them biologically active. Perhaps pure iodine has a similar action to thyroid hormones, but you just need more of it? What gave me the clue for this idea was a colleague's patient who had had a total thyroidectomy for cancer. Blood tests showed extremely low levels of thyroid hormone but clinically she was normal (euthyroid). She had achieved such by taking

---

‡**Archaeological note:** 'Omo I' refers to a collection of hominin bones (classified anatomically as modern humans (Homo sapiens)) discovered between 1967 and 1974 at sites near the Omo River, in south-western Ethiopia; these are East Africa's oldest human remains and recently they have been dated as being even older than first thought. They are now dated at 233,000 years old, 36,000 years older than previously thought.[24]

large doses of iodine which she was using for its anticancer properties.

We have a medical precedent for this. Jean-Francois Coindet (1774 – 1834, Swiss physician and researcher) in 1820 used up to 250 mg iodine a day in order to successfully treat goitre (from the Latin *gutturia*, meaning throat) – the classic neck swelling that develops with long-term underactive thyroid as the thyroid gland enlarges to try to make up for the deficit. In other words, he reversed hypothyroidism with generous doses of iodine.

Coindet used three different preparations, a solution of potassium iodide, an iodide-iodine solution somewhat different from the one that Lugol later defined, and an alcoholic (tincture) solution that Coindet later was to recommend as the safest and easiest to use. Twenty drops of these solutions contained approximately 50 mg (one 'French grain') of iodine. Coindet routinely prescribed 10 drops three times a day for the first week (75 mg), and then 15 drops thrice a day for the second week (112 mg) and 20 drops three times a day (150 mg) subsequently. He only rarely prescribed higher doses. The recommended duration of treatment was 8-10 weeks. Results of the treatment were spectacular: softening and shrinking of goitres occurred after 8 days, and disappearance or a significant improvement in disfiguring or uncomfortable goitres occurred later in many cases. In addition, he observed iodine had a general stimulating effect on the appetite, the uterus, acted as an aphrodisiac, and he concluded that, used with competence, iodine would become one of the most potent medications brought to medicine by modern chemistry.[25]

Not only was Coindet shrinking goitres, but the stimulating aphrodisiac effects suggest he was improving energy delivery mechanisms by reversing hypothyroidism.

It may be that with application of all the principles detailed in this book, those needing thyroid glandular can gradually tail off its use. Should such an experiment be tried, it must be done very slowly and monitored carefully with symptoms, signs and blood tests. Watch this space!

Appendices

Appendix A

How to access thyroid blood tests

The bare minimum testing you need to get started is a TSH, free T4 and free T3. These are readily available to all doctors. The problem is that many doctors do not appreciate the need for all three. This is particularly the case when they only recognise primary thyroid disease and ignore secondary hypothyroidism, poor T4 to T3 conversion and thyroid hormone receptor resistance, as described in Chapter 1.

Thyroid hormones are stable in the bloodstream and so these tests can be done on postal samples. In addition, only small volumes of blood are required and so tests can be readily done on a DIY finger-prick sample of blood. You can do these yourself at home with no need for a nurse to draw blood.

Labs that accept such samples in the UK can be found at the relevant webpage of Natural Health Worldwide here: https://naturalhealthworldwide.com/lab-tests/. Such labs include:

* Medichecks – for example, this test covers thyroid antibodies, free T3, free T4 and TSH: https://medichecks.com/products/thyroid-function-antibodies-blood-test
* Medichecks – for example, this test covers free T3, free T4 and TSH: https://medichecks.com/products/thyroid-function-blood-test
* Thriva – for example, this test covers vitamins D and B12, ferritin, thyroid antibodies, free T3, free T4 and TSH: https://thriva.co/blood-test-packages/thyroid-blood-test
* PrivateBloodTests – https://privatebloodtests.co.uk/pages/thyroid-blood-tests

Thyroid UK is a very helpful charity and I recommend that you use their resources:

- for general information: https://thyroiduk.org/
- for private blood tests:
  https://thyroiduk.org/help-and-support/private-thyroid-tests-in-the-uk/

You can source help from practitioners at Natural Health Worldwide (https://natural-healthworldwide.com/) and there is a list of mobile phlebotomists, if needed, on that website (https://naturalhealthworldwide.com/mobile-phlebotomists/). Contact the labs directly for costs, kits and packaging.

Appendix B

The different thyroid glandular preparations and how to obtain them

For a list of standardised, licensed, medicinal, natural desiccated thyroid (NDT) preparations see https://thyroiduk.org/if-you-are-hypothyroid/medication-for-hypothyroidism/. These include brands such as Armour thyroid, Thyroid-S, Westhroid, Nature-Throid, Erfa, WP Thyroid and NP thyroid, with doses classically measured in 'grains'.

Wholefood desiccated thyroid (WDT), also called 'thyroid glandular', is the original and the best preparation, because being unmodified and non-standardised, it is the most physiological and natural form of these dried meats. It comes in milligram sizing, and can be obtained from many food supplement company sources. It is available from pork and from beef sources.

In my experience, one grain of NDT is approximately equivalent to 60 mg of pork glandular and 65 mg of beef glandular. Most people (depending on their body weight) end up on 60-120 mg of pork glandular or 65-130 mg of beef glandular (see Chapter 6).

Table B.1: NDT/thyroid glandular preparations

NDT product	Ingredients	Approx cost at time of going to press
Allergy Research Group Thyroid Natural Glandular www.allergyresearchgroup.com	Thyroid (40 mg bovine, lyophilised/freeze-dried from New Zealand/Australia), hydroxypropyl methylcellulose, microcrystalline cellulose, L-leucine	Works out to about $4.44 per gram of WDT

Table B.1 (cont'd)

NDT product	Ingredients	Approx cost at time of going to press
Ancestral Supplements Grassfed Beef Thyroid www.ancestralsupplements.com	Freeze-dried New Zealand grass-fed desiccated beef thyroid with liver (30 mg thyroid, 470 mg liver), collagen (bovine gelatin) capsules	Works out to about $8.52 per gram of WDT
Dr. Ron's Ultra-Pure Thyroid With Liver www.drrons.com	Freeze-dried New Zealand thyroid (bovine, 30 mg per capsule), freeze-dried New Zealand liver (bovine), New Zealand bovine gelatin capsules	Works out to about $11.10 per gram of WDT
ForefrontHealth Raw Desiccated Thyroid www.forefronthealth.com	Raw desiccated New Zealand bovine thyroid (65 mg or 130 mg depending on product), rice flour, cellulose, dicalcium phosphate, silica, gelatin, purified water. ForeforntHealth says, 'processed by low temperature lyophilization to ensure and preserve natural constituents'	Works out to about $2.56 per gram of WDT with the 130 mg version
Natural Sources Raw Thyroid www.vitacost.com	Thyroid tissue (50 mg, freeze-dried), adrenal tissue (20 mg), pituitary tissue (10 mg), thymus tissue (5 mg), spleen tissue (4 mg), capsule (gelatin), magnesium stearate (vegetable source), kelp (probably included to add iodine), flogard (a precipitated silica flow/anti-caking agent)	Works out to about $3.03 per gram of WDT
Natural Thyroid Solutions Thyro-Gold www.naturalthyroidsolutions Two dosages available – 150 mg and 300 mg. The manufacturer says the 300 mg is designed only for people whose thyroid has been removed, and suggests avoiding more than two 300 mg capsules without 'the guidance and care of a qualified clinician'	Whole-gland thyroid powder from pasture-fed New Zealand cattle, L-aspartic acid, Coleus Forskohlii, vegetable capsules (probably hydroxypropyl methylcellulose), silica, certified organic coconut oil powder	Works out to about $2.35 per gram of WDT

NuMedica Thyrodex T-150 www.vitacost.com	Vitamin A (as beta carotene), riboflavin (vitamin B2), calcium (as calcium citrate and calcium bisglycinate chelate), iodine (from kelp, 400 mcg), magnesium (as magnesium oxide), zinc (as zinc citrate and zinc bisglycinate chelate), manganese (as manganese citrate and manganese bisglycinate chelate), potassium (as potassium gluconate hydrochloride), thyroid tissue (bovine, 150 mg), L-tyrosine, Irish moss seaweed (Chondrus crispus), parsley (Petroselinum crispum, leaf), adrenal gland (tissue, bovine), pituitary (tissue, bovine), horsetail (Equisetum arvense), spleen (tissue, bovine), rice flour, hydroxypropyl methylcellulose (vegetable capsule), magnesium stearate	Works out to about $3.32 per gram of WDT
Nutri-Meds Desiccated Thyroid www.nutri-meds.com	Has historically been available in a choice of bovine or porcine, although the porcine is currently not listed on the website. The remaining ingredients in the capsule version are gelatin from free-range sources, L-Leucine, L-Lysine and silica. For the tablet version they are dicalcium phosphate (as a binder) and pharmaceutical glaze (for easier swallowing). Nutri-Meds say, 'tissue processed by the Low Temperature Method to preserve natural constituents'	Works out to about $2.82 per gram of WDT
Procepts Nutrition Metavive I, II, III, IV (UK product) www.the-natural-choice. co.uk - Metavive I (porcine thyroid complex 40 mg) and - Metavive II (porcine thyroid complex 80 mg)	Rice bran, porcine thyroid complex (standardised 5'-ribonucleotides, porcine thyroid gland), vegetable cellulose capsule. The pigs are born outdoors and raised hormone/antibiotic-free. The thyroids are freeze-dried and low-temperature processed	Prices can be seen at www.the-natural-choice. co.uk
- Metavive III (bovine thyroid complex 40 mg) and - Metavive IV (bovine thyroid complex 80 mg)	Rice bran, bovine thyroid complex (bovine thyroid gland, standardised 5'-ribonucleotides), vegetable cellulose capsule. The cows are raised hormone/antibiotic-free and are outdoor/pasture-raised. The thyroids are freeze-dried and low-temperature processed	Prices can be seen at www.the-natural-choice. co.uk

Appendix C

The paleo-ketogenic (PK) diet

Why a PK diet and how to get into ketosis
Balancing up calories, protein and carbs
Fasting

The cure is in the kitchen.

Dr Sherry Rogers, environmental physician

The paleo-ketogenic (PK) diet is non-negotiable in maintaining and restoring health. It is the starting point to treat every disease. I spend more time talking about diet and cooking than all other subjects put together. Changing one's diet is the most difficult but the most important thing one needs to do for good health. There is much more detail of the Why and the How in our books *Prevent and cure Diabetes: delicious diets not dangerous drugs* and *Paleo-Ketogenic: The Why and the How*. Please do use them – they are born out of bitter experience. However, the key aim is to use ketones (from fats and fermented fibre) rather than glucose to power our cells as this is the preferred food/energy source for our mitochondria – the power-generators in our cells that turn said food into the energy currency on which our bodies run, ATP (adenosine triphosphate). And it has been for millions of years. If any sugar, or carbohydrate that can be turned into sugar, is available our bodies will use that as the easy option. Hence, to put ourselves in 'ketosis' (fat burning rather than sugar burning) we need to eat very little carbohydrate and replace this with fats as our energy source.

Remember, outside autumn primitive man ate a paleo-ketogenic diet and this would be largely comprised of raw meat and/or raw fish and shellfish, depending on where he lived. That was it. You might think this a boring diet, but boredom is secondary to survival. For some of the sickest patients, we have to return to this primitive carnivore diet to allow them to recover – this is based on meat, fish and eggs. An essential part of this diet is to access bone marrow. Perhaps this is what drove primitive man to using tools to smash open this treasure chest of fat and micronutrients and so the clever ones survived? Neanderthal man had a larger brain than modern man.

As my patients often hear in the consulting room: 'My job is to get you well, not to entertain you.' I repeat this in all our books. (Some say that quoting oneself lacks humility. It is a good job then that Craig wrote that last paragraph.)

Guess what? I am not going to live my life eating raw meat and raw fish just so that I can live to a great age. We all have to work out a compromise diet that gets the best of both worlds. And that is going to be different for everyone and will change with age. For me, greed gets in the way – I love good food! So, we all need a starting point which can then be relaxed or tightened up depending on age and disease state. Younger, healthy, physically active people can take more liberties than old, sick ones. I find myself in the old, healthy category and so I am still no paragon of virtue.

What to eat to get into ketosis

A reasonable starting point for most is the following, divided into: (1) foods you can eat any amount of because they contain no carbs; (2) foods that are less than 5% carb; (3) foods to take care with but not because of carbs; (4) foods with which care is needed because they contain 5-10% carbs; and (5) foods that contain more than 10% carbs so should be avoided.

1. No-carb foods you can eat as much of as you like

•   Fats: Saturated fats for energy, such as lard, butter and ideally ghee (so long as you are sure you are not allergic to dairy; I am… dammit), goose fat, coconut oil, palm oil.

- Oils: Unsaturated fats which are also fuels but contain essential omega-3 and omega-6 plus omega-9 fatty acids. Hemp oil is ideal, containing the perfect proportion of omega-6 to omega-3 – that is, 4:1. These must be cold-pressed and not used for cooking or you risk 'flipping' them into toxic trans fats. Only cook with biochemically stable, saturated fats. (See Glossary, page 184-186, for more on good and bad fats.)
- Fibre: This is often included in the carb count of foods and leads to some confusion. Eat enough fibre for you to be crapping like one of Denis Burkitt's Africans. Burkitt, consultant surgeon, observed that indigenous Africans did not suffer Western diseases. For these Africans, normal defaecation meant twice daily squatting to produce a turd effortlessly (no straining), cucumber-size, no cracks, no balling, soft and inoffensive. To be precise, type 4 on the Bristol stool chart. To achieve that which colorectal surgeons dream of you need to consume half a PK loaf daily (see *Paleo-Ketogenic: The Why and the How*) or its fibre equivalent. Then invest in a squatty potty – I was delighted to read that some have 'motion sensitive lights'. Consuming a high-fibre diet also means that fermentation of fibre in the large bowel generates vitamin K.

2. Foods that have less than 5% carb

The most important of these are:
- Linseed: *Paleo-Ketogenic: The Why and the How* has a great recipe for linseed bread which looks and behaves like a small Hovis; linseed also makes a great base for muesli and porridge. These days I find making buns quicker than a loaf; they cook reliably well in 40 minutes at 220°C. Fashion the dough into a rolling pin shape and cut out 12 discs.
- Coconut cream: The Grace coconut milk is head and shoulders above all others with a 2% carb content. It is a great dairy alternative.
- Brazil and pecan nuts.
- Salad (lettuce, cucumber, tomato, pepper etc); avocado pear and olives (phew! I love them both).
- Green leafy vegetables.
- Mushrooms and fungi: A difficulty with the PK diet is eating enough fat. These foods

are great for frying as they mop up delicious, saturated fats.
- Fermented foods (sauerkraut, kefir): The carb content has been fermented out by microbes.

3. Non-carb foods to take care with for other reasons

There are other reasons to take care with:
- Meat, fish, shellfish and eggs: Do not consume too much as excessive amounts can be converted back to carbohydrate in a process called gluconeogenesis (see *Paleo-Ketogenic: The Why and the How* for details).
- Salt: 1 tsp (5 g) daily. Ideally use Sunshine salt as below.
- Coffee and tea: Drink in moderation.

4. Foods that are 5-10% carb

Foods that are 5-10% carb can be included in moderation. There is much more detail in *Paleo-Ketogenic: The Why and the How* but these are the most important:
- Berries.
- Some nuts: Almonds.
- Herbs and spices: These do have a carb content, but in the small amounts normally used these are not going to spike sugar levels.

5. Foods that are more than 10% carb

Foods that are more than 10% carb are to be avoided as they switch on addictive eating. (I know – I too am an addict!) These foods include:
- All grains, pulses, fruit (apart from berries) and their juices.
- Many nuts and seeds: Pistachios.
- Junk food, which is characterised by its high-carb content and additive potential.
- All dairy products except ghee.

Avoid all sweeteners, natural or artificial, as they simply switch on the physical and psychological craving.

Ensuring you are in ketosis

Ketones arise through burning fat as your energy source and their presence indicates that you are successfully achieving this through your PK diet. Fat burning generates three types of ketone that can be tested for to see how you are doing:

- Beta-hydroxybutyric acid: This is present in, and can be measured in, the blood; it is the most accurate measure, but testing strips are expensive. I am mean and also a wimp, so I do not use this method.
- Acetoacetate: This is excreted in the urine. Testing is cheap and easy with urine keto-stix but as the body becomes more efficient at matching ketone production to demand, urine tests may show false negatives.
- Acetone: This is exhaled and can be measured with breath testing. This is my preferred method as you can easily test after every meal to ensure you have not overdone the carbs. You will need to invest in a breath meter to do this.

Trouble-shooting the ketone breath test

If your diet is sufficiently low-carb, expect to blow 2-4 parts per million (ppm) of ketones. However, as I have said, the body will always use sugar in preference to ketones. This means that *any* amount of ketones in your breath signifies that you are in ketosis provided there is no contamination involved (see next).

If you blow very high ketones – say up to 10 ppm – this may be for one of these reasons:

- When stressed, there is an outpouring of adrenalin and this stimulates fat burning.
- Over-dosing with thyroid hormones may cause high levels of ketones.
- Fasting: Even on a PK diet you consume some carbohydrates. With fasting you get *all* your calories from fat, so ketones are higher. This illustrates the point that even in mild ketosis you will be using some sugars as a fuel; that is fine.
- Contamination as below.

You can get **false positive** results:

- The mechanism used to measure ketones is the same as that for measuring alcohol. You may see a positive if: you have consumed any alcohol in the past 24 hours (depending on how much!).

- If you have an upper fermenting gut (see page 187), then this too produces alcohol.
- Any products containing alcohol may give a positive result. I checked this myself with an alcohol wipe (often used for hand sanitising) to clean the mouthpiece and this gave a high reading.
- The breath meter measures parts per million – it is very sensitive. You only need a tiny amount of contaminant to upset the result. Many household cleaners contain volatile organic compounds which may register on the meter.

Other possible issues

- You can also get **false negative** results. If you have anything to eat or drink in the preceding 20 minutes then that may affect the test. For example, I know if I have a sip of coffee then that may be followed by a negative reading.
- The actual figure may not reflect blood levels of ketones. This is partly because blood ketones are different – they are beta-hydroxybutyric acid (see above) whereas breath ketones are acetones.
- The result may not square with urine ketones. Again, this is because urine ketones are different (acetoacetate). It is common to see ketones on a breath test, but the urine test be negative for the reasons given above – with time, the body gets better at matching energy demands to delivery, so fewer ketones are 'wasted' through urinary losses.

Is being in ketosis safe?

Being in ketosis is *not* dangerous but most doctors do not understand this. They do not know about or understand physiological ketosis. They only know about diabetic ketoacidosis and may panic if you tell them you are in ketosis.

When ketosis is a problem

Ketosis is *only* a medical problem if you are diabetic and your blood sugars are running high (either because your medication is insufficient *or* you are consuming too many carbs). For example, a blood sugar above 10 mmol/l and/or the presence of sugar in your urine IS A MEDICAL EMERGENCY.

Bear in mind that the DIY home tests for blood sugar rely on a test that employs glucose oxidase. Vitamin C cross-reacts – so if you are taking vitamin C to bowel tolerance, as recommended in this book, your blood will be saturated with vitamin C and this may give false highs. My experience is that this may be 2-3 mmol/l higher than the actual blood glucose. That is to say an apparent reading of 7-8 mol/l equates to a real reading of 4-5 mmol/l of glucose.

Balancing up total calories, protein and carbs

Having established ketosis, you need to balance up total calories, protein and carbs.

Calories

The total calories you need per day will depend on your age, weight, height and activity. You can look this up here: www.calculator.net/calorie-calculator.html. Your calorie requirement *at rest* is often referred to as your 'basal metabolic rate' (BMR). Knowing this is essential for calculating your overall calorie needs – see below for how to determine both.

Do not regularly eat less than your daily calorie requirement or your body will simply switch off calorie burning to make you tired, foggy, cold and depressed (but see intermittent fasting below).

Protein

Protein sources include meat, eggs, fish and shellfish. These are zero carb *but*, if eaten in excess, the body can convert them into sugars. A rule of thumb is to allow 0.7 to 0.9 grams (g) of protein per pound (0.45 kg) of lean body mass, but see below for protein leverage.

The PK diet is not a high-protein diet. It is high in fat and fibre (relative to Western diets). Fibre is important to satisfy the appetite. The key is to eat no refined or heavily processed foods and calculate your protein needs.

Your protein needs – not too little, not too much: Protein leverage

The body cannot store protein, but daily protein is essential for survival. We have a protein appetite which will make us crave food until that appetite has been satisfied. If you are eating a low-protein diet, you will be driven to eat more food. In that process you are likely to over-eat carbs and fat and so expect to gain weight. Conversely, eat a high-protein diet and you tend to under-eat and lose weight. It is therefore important to get your protein intake right to help maintain a normal weight. For this you need to know your BMR. (Note a high-protein diet is also not desirable as the body then has to deal with the toxic consequences of too much protein. Listen to your body and appetite; they will tell you how much you need.)

Calculating your calorie requirement
1. Calculating your basal metabolic rate (BMR)

First you need to calculate your calorie needs at rest (your BMR). There are many equations to do this; we shall be using a tried-and-tested formula, the Mifflin – St Jeor equations which are:

> For men: 10 x Weight (kg) PLUS 6.25 x Height (cm) MINUS 5 x Age (years) PLUS 5

> For women: 10 x Weight (kg) PLUS 6.25 x Height (cm) MINUS 5 x Age (years) MINUS 161

If you'd rather not do the maths, this handy online calculator does it for you: www.calculator.net/bmr-calculator.html

2. Calculating your total daily calorie requirement

Then to calculate your total daily calorie requirement you will need to multiply up your BMR by these factors depending on your level of activity. Again, the website above does this for you:

Sedentary:	calories required = BMR x 1.2
Lightly active:	calories required = BMR x 1.375
Moderately active (moderate exercise 3-5 days):	calories required = BMR x 1.55

Very active   calories required = BMR x 1.725
(hard exercise 6-7 days a week):

Super active   calories required = BMR x 1.9
(hard exercise and sport and physical job):

Table C.1 shows a worked example (based on me) and Figure C.1 is a screenshot of the same calculation done via the bmr-calculator link. You can see that the BMR of 1189 kcal and total energy expenditure of 1843 kcal (Figure C.1) agree with my calculated figures in Table C.1.

Table C.1: Calorie needs at rest (BMR) and when active, with worked example

Steps FIRST work out your BMR at rest	Worked example – My vital statistics are: weight 61 kg height 168 cm age 62 Result for me	
For women: BMR = 10 x weight (kg) PLUS 6.25 x height (cm) minus 5 x age (years) MINUS 161	10 x 61 kg = 610 PLUS 6.25 x 168 cm = 1050 MINUS 5 x 62 = 310 MINUS 161	610 PLUS 1050 MINUS 310 MINUS 161 My BMR is 1189 kcal
For men: BMR = 10 x weight (kg) PLUS 6.25 x height (cm) MINUS 5 x age (years) PLUS 5	Ditto above THEN ADD 5	If I were male, and Craig says I do have balls, the calculation would be: 610 PLUS 1050 MINUS 310 PLUS 5 My BMR would be 1355 kcal

Steps FIRST work out your BMR at rest	Worked example – My vital statistics are: weight 61 kg height 168 cm age 62 Result for me	
THEN multiply your resting BMR by your activity factor to get your total energy expenditure: • Sedentary x 1.2 • Lightly active x 1.375 • Moderately active (moderate exercise 3-5 days) x 1.55 • Very active (hard exercise 6-7 days a week) x 1.725 • Super-active (hard exercise and sport and physical job) x 1.9	I am moderately active so I: MULTIPLY my BMR by a factor of 1.55 = 1189 x 1.55 = 1843	So my daily energy expenditure is 1843 kcal

Figure C.1: Screenshot of the calculation in Table C.1 done using the link www.calculator.net/bmr-calculator.html

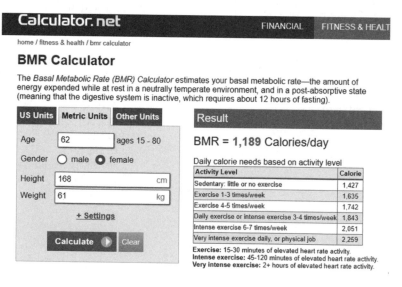

Calculating your daily protein requirement

Table C.2 then shows how to calculate your daily protein requirement and Table C.3 shows how to meet that need in terms of actual foods.

Table C.2: How to calculate your protein requirement

Steps	Worked example – me	Result for me
FIRST work out your daily energy expenditure as above	My daily energy expenditure is 1843 kcal	
Then divide by 4 to give your daily protein need in grams (this need includes recycled protein from self)	DIVIDE 1843 by 4 = 461	
Then adjust for age protein requirements as % of daily energy requirement • Baby to adolescent: 15% • Young adult to 30 years: 18% • Pregnancy and breast-feeding: 20% • 30s: 17% • 40-60: 15% • 60-65: 18% • >65: 20%	I am 62 so I need my diet to be 18% protein 461 x 18/100 = 83	So, I need 83 grams of protein daily

Once you have things roughly balanced out, your body will do the rest. Appetite and desire for food are remarkably accurate once you have addiction out of the way. Interestingly, before I did this calculation what's listed in Table C.3 was what I ate, so my brain and body had worked it out already.

Table C.3: What and how much to eat to satisfy your protein requirement

Food	Protein content in grams (g) per 100 g	On the plate looks like... approx.	What I eat	My protein consumption approx
Eggs	13	Two eggs	Breakfast: 2 eggs	13
Beef	26	A medium beef burger		
Pork	31	Small pork chop	Supper, main course: pork chop	31
Bacon	Up to 39 depending on how fatty; 1 slice = 8 g			
Lamb	26	One lamb chop		
Chicken, duck	20	Whole breast or Whole leg		
Fish, fresh	29	A good chunk		
Prawns	25	A prawn 'cocktail' starter	Supper, starters: pate or fish	25
Brazil nuts	15		Snacks	10-15
				My total: 79-84

Establishing the PK diet

If the PK diet really does not suit you in the short term, this may be due to a DDD (detox or die-ff) reaction (see Appendix G).

If it really does not suit you in the long term there may be other reasons. We do know that sugar is a vital part of metabolism – NOT as a fuel, but as a building block to make DNA and RNA. It is also essential for detoxing via the glucuronide pathway in the liver.

I think the most important information is that being in ketosis tells us our glycogen stores are squeezed dry. At this point, consuming some carbs is fine – if you slip out of ketosis for a short time then you are doing no harm. I am sometimes out of ketosis in the morning, but by late afternoon I am invariably blowing ketones.

Sugars may come from protein (via gluconeogenesis) or, of course, from eating carbs. Low-protein and zero-carb diets are not desirable, for all the reasons given.

If you really struggle to get into ketosis, then I suggest a 5:2 diet – that is, you eat the best low-carb you can manage for five days, then for two days a week you eat a *very* low-carb diet, or possibly fast until you get into ketosis. The important point here is that to get into ketosis you have to squeeze dry the glycogen 'sponges' in the liver and muscle. Once these stores have been emptied, blood sugar control is much easier as the body is not relying on insulin and this avoids high blood sugar, and the blood sugar swings of metabolic syndrome.

REMEMBER THE ABOVE ARE NOT HARD AND FAST RULES – LISTEN TO YOUR BODY AND FOLLOW YOUR APPETITE. ONCE YOU ARE NOT ADDICTED TO FOODS SUCH AS CARBS AND SUGAR THIS IS A REMARKABLY GOOD GUIDE!

Variety is the very spice of life, that gives it all its flavour.
William Cowper's poem *The Task*, 1785

Change your diet with the seasons and through life. With your food addictions gone, eat foods that you enjoy most because these will be the very foods that you need. A wide variety of foods will grow a wide variety of microbes in the gut. Include as many spices and herbs as you can. Taste has evolved for excellent reasons! Eat foods that have had very little processing. Become a gardener and grow your own, even if you only have a window box.

And if you have decided to go ahead with this diet, then believe me it is a bumpy ride. There is a whole new language to be learned. You will have to identify the glycogen sponge, anticipate the metabolic hinterland, get keto-adapted and prepare for detox and Herx reactions (see Appendix G). I simply cannot write all the nitty gritty detail here for this successful transition without losing the plot of this book... at least get *Paleo-Ketogenic: The Why and the How* which holds your intellectual hand through this difficult transition. Or just do it...

Supplements and the PK diet

We need supplementary vitamins and minerals simply because, with Western agriculture, there is a one-way movement of minerals from the soil to plants, to animals and then to us humans. We throw them away. This lack of recycling means we are all deficient. Once again, we discuss this in much more detail in our book *Paleo-Ketogenic: The Why and the How*, with referenced studies showing the result of this 'one-way' traffic.

I have got to the stage of my medicine where I know exactly what must be done so I am now trying to make this as easy and inexpensive as possible. So, I have put together 'Sunshine Salt' which contains all the essential minerals, from sodium and selenium to magnesium and manganese, together with vitamin D 5000 iu and vitamin B12 5 mg per 5-gram (1-tsp) dose. This does make life much easier. It tastes like a slightly piquant sea salt, can be used in cooking and means the rest of the family get a dose without realising it, especially that man* who believes he is immortal.

In addition, we all need vitamin C: 5-15 grams (yes I mean 5000 to 15,000 mg, and no, that is not a big dose) daily (see Appendices D and E for the How plus our book *The Infection Game* for the Why).

Timing – when to eat

Primitive man did not eat three regular meals a day, neither did he snack. Consultant neurologist Dale Bredesen reverses dementia with a PK diet but insists all daily food is consumed within a 10-hour window of time.[1]

Once keto-adapted you may feel a bit peckish and deserving of a snack, but the good news is that you will not get the associated 'energy dive' experienced by the carb addict who must eat according to the clock. Carb addicts feel a sudden loss of energy and *have* to feed their addiction to get rid of this awful feeling. The keto-adapted do not experience this.

---

*Aside from Craig, born a man, having had honorary womanhood bestowed upon him: It is a shame that 'ichor' (the 'blood' of the Greek Gods which was said to retain the qualities of ambrosia, the food or drink of the gods, which gave them immortality) does not seem to exist. And so, until ichor is found, or formulated, and made non-toxic to mortals, I shall 'eat PK', take my supplements and openly sprinkle Sunshine Salt over my food.

A weekly 24-hour fast is also good for the metabolism (see next). It may be counter-intuitive, but the fact is that this enhances mental and physical performance.

The word doctor comes from the Latin to teach. I can show you the path, but you have to walk it. You have to become your own doctor. All diagnosis starts with hypothesis. We know the PK diet is the starting point to treat every disease and that is non-negotiable. Stick with this diet for life and it may be that this is all you have to do. Once PK is established you have to ask if you are functioning to your full physical and mental potential? Only you can know this.

If you are functioning to your full potential, then you can take the occasional liberty with your diet. Primitive man surely did. He did so in the autumn, although not with the high-carb foods that we can now access. Alcohol is a peculiar problem – it is addictive, high-carb and stimulates insulin directly. But I love alcohol – the jokes are so much funnier with a glass of cider on board and so I enjoy this occasional liberty at this stage in my life.

If you are not functioning to your full potential, then you must stick with the PK diet. Even if you do not experience immediate benefits you will greatly increase your chance of a long and healthy life. It is a great consolation for me to be able to tell my CFS and ME patients that their best years are ahead of them.

Fasting – a great therapeutic tool

Primitive man feasted and fasted. So do all carnivores. It makes perfect evolutionary sense that to fast enhances physical and mental performance – it made Man a better hunter. He got hungry for food… and we use this very word to describe the will and energy to succeed. Mozart produced his finest works when hungry for money, as did Van Gogh and Dickens. Being hungry enhances performance.

> *Fasting is the first principle of medicine: fast and see the strength of the spirit reveal itself.*
>
> Rumi (1207 – 1273)
> 13th-century Persian, poet, faqih, Islamic scholar, theologian and Sufi mystic, originally from Greater Khorasan in Greater Iran

Fasting has many benefits, including for weight loss, lowering blood pressure and cholesterol, restoring insulin sensitivity, fighting infection, detoxification, cell repair ('autophagy') and enhancing performance. It is the most inexpensive therapeutic tool, it multitasks as below, and the potential for side-effects or harm is miniscule. I like that sort of medicine! When I fast the usual chores of shopping, cooking, washing up and clearing away vanish. I have more time and energy for all else. I have now come to joyfully anticipate my fasts.

Promotes weight loss

We know calorie restriction does not work. It is easy to see why – prolonged mild starvation results in the body shutting down energy expenditure. This makes us physically tired, brain-dead and depressed. The body quickly matches energy spending to energy delivery, so weight loss ceases but we remain fat, fatigued, foggy and in a funk hole. The answer is to take advantage of the inherent, metabolic inertia that means it takes several days for our metabolism to slow. Eat your normal PK diet for five days then fast for two. You continue to burn fat at your normal rate throughout, so mental and physical energy remain normal, but your weekly calorie consumption is reduced by 2/7ths (28%).

Fat comes off the belly first – this is because when fasting there can be no gut fermentation and fat is dumped where the immune system is busy as it demands a lot of energy.

The modern fad to treat obesity is bariatric surgery (252,000 operations in USA 2018). Yes, it works for weight loss, but health losses include: dumping syndrome, malnutrition, vomiting, ulcers, bowel obstruction, hernia, blood clots, gallstones and more. Fasting is more effective and a darn sight safer.

Reverses hypertension and high cholesterol

Both blood pressure and cholesterol normalise on a PK diet. Fasting makes this happen more quickly. If they do not normalise, look for other causes such as high homocysteine, thyroid problems (as described in the rest of this book!) and sleep disturbance.

Restores insulin sensitivity

Insulin resistance is the hallmark of type 2 diabetes. If not already in ketosis, fasting empties glycogen stores, reverses insulin resistance and is the fastest way to lose weight, reverse metabolic syndrome and diabetes. Diabetics and their doctors are naturally anxious about low blood sugar. This can *only* happen if the diabetic is taking prescribed medication to lower blood sugar. The key is to monitor blood sugar closely and, as levels come down as they inevitably will, reduce the dose of medication. Type 2 diabetics should be able to stop all medication. Type 1 diabetics *must* use continuous blood sugar monitoring such as Dexcom. They eventually need a smaller dose of insulin, and a few will end up on no insulin. The 'brittle' diabetics are stabilised.

As I've said earlier in this Appendix, doctors always fret about their patients being in ketosis because the only state they know about is diabetic ketoacidosis – a dire emergency. Diabetic ketoacidosis occurs when blood sugar is very high. This problem is entirely preventable with careful blood sugar monitoring, and note my advice above (page 127) regarding vitamin C's effect on blood sugar measurement.

Enhances performance

Human growth hormone spikes with fasting; this results in more muscle being laid down (so we can run faster and throw those primitive spears further) together with fat burning. Metabolic rate increases by up to 14%. Again, we see that fasting enhances performance – the Samurai warrior fasted before fighting. Indeed, before battle, the Samurai warrior was advised to drink only 'hot water that had been poured over rice'.[†]

Restores thyroid sensitivity?

I suspect, but do not yet know, that fasting also improves thyroid hormone receptor resistance, perhaps for the same reason it reverses insulin hormone receptor resistance. I say this because I have now seen several patients able to reduce their daily dose of thyroid hormone with fasting regimes.

Treats infections

All infections, including viral, are fed by sugar. Fasting and rest mean all energy is available for the immune system to fight the good fight.

> *Fast a cold, fast a fever.*
> Old adage,
> Myhill adapted, with apologies

[†]**Footnote:** This quotation is from *The Hundred Rules of War* by Tsukahara Bokuden, 1489 – 1571. Interested readers can still buy this book from Amazon among other sources. For film buffs, the scene from the *Seven Samurai*, in which the character Gorobei's swordsmanship skills are tested is based on an episode from Tsukahara's life.

Detoxifies

The greatest source of toxic stress in the body comes from the gut. Obviously fasting greatly reduces this burden.

Fat is a repository for fat-soluble toxins – see Appendix G for DDD reactions. Fasting mobilises toxins PDQ (pretty damn quick!) which can then be excreted.

Allows autophagy (literally 'self-eating')

When fuel and raw materials do not come through from the gut, the body looks to itself for these. It finds energy initially from liver and muscle glycogen stores (about 2000 kcal – so the non-keto marathon runners get to 17 miles before 'hitting a wall'), then by fat burning. Protein cannot be stored, so the body obtains such from recycling old, worn out cells. This is the metabolic equivalent of spring cleaning and it has profoundly beneficial effects. So-called autophagy has anti-inflammatory, rejuvenating, anti-cancer and healing properties. Indeed, for thousands of years fasting has been used to treat an alphabet of disease: arterial disease and arthritis, brain tumours, cancer, dementia, epilepsy, fatigue, hypertension, gastritis, Hodgkin's and more.

> *Fasting is the greatest remedy - the physician within.*
> *Paracelsus, 5th century Swiss-German Renaissance physician and botanist*

Stimulates cell growth

Fasting shifts stem cells from a dormant state to a state of self-renewal so it is good for:
- The immune system: old cells are killed off and young front-line fighters grown.
- The brain: neurones make more connections.
- The rest of the body: new young cells for the gut, liver, skin, blood vessels, connective tissue, heart, muscle and bone.

Treats cancer

We know the ketogenic diet starves cancer cells of sugar, without which they cannot be fuelled. Fasting increases ketosis even more – combine this with the immune stimulation of fasting and vitamin C to bowel tolerance and, yes, you are really winning!

Autophagy digests cancer cells too. Fasting before and during chemotherapy enhances the effects of treatment and minimises side effects and it also enhances the effects of radiotherapy. I would recommend fasting on the day before and the day of such treatments, possibly longer.

Dr Thomas Seyfried, consultant oncologist, reckons we should all to an annual fast of one week to substantially reduce the incidence of all cancers.

Treats dementia

Consultant neurologist Dr Dale Bredesen has reversed dementia with a ketogenic diet in many patients. Fasting does this faster. Remember foggy brain is an early symptom of dementia!

How to fast

Preparation includes:
- Get keto-adapted first. This avoids many of the DDD reactions (Appendix G) which are an inevitable result of getting into ketosis.
- Anticipate:
  - Social opprobrium – When I announced I was going to do a five-day fast, my friends were immediately anxious for my physical and mental health!
  - Fear of hunger, and accompanying such, fear of fatigue and fear of foggy brain.

However, as you will discover, there is nothing to fear and, with time and practice, you will look forward to your fasts. Hunger is greatly ameliorated by telling your brain that you are going to do it regardless of its nagging. You make your mind up and feel proud that you can do what all others fear.

> *In the afternoon, the digestion of the meal deprives me of the incomparable lightness which characterizes the fast days.*
> Adalbert De Vogue, 1924 – 2011, Benedictine monk

> *I fast for greater physical and mental efficiency.*
> Plato, 424/423 – 348/347 BC, who was taught by Socrates and who taught Aristotle.

What you do consume

Yes, you must drink water and take electrolytes. The ideal mix is spring water with Sunshine Salt. Whilst one can drink pure water you cannot sweat or pee pure water –

both sweat and pee contain minerals, not just sodium chloride (table salt) but all, from magnesium and molybdenum to calcium and chromium. Sunshine Salt provides every permitted essential mineral in the correct physiological proportions. This makes for the perfect hydration mix – 5 grams of Sunshine Salt per one litre of water, drunk according to thirst.

Carry on your usual nutritional supplements, including vitamin C at least 5 grams or to bowel tolerance.

If you are on prescription medication, carry on but monitor effects. The need for most comes down, especially drugs for hypertension (check BP daily), diabetes (monitor blood sugar), asthma (check peak flow), painkillers, anti-inflammatories and, I suspect, thyroid hormones!

Do not confuse hunger pangs with greed or need. Use hot water and lemon juice to postpone the 'breakthrough' waves of hunger, and by the time you are sipping you will find that the wave has passed.

How long to fast

If you are in good health:

- Start by eating all your PK meals within a 10-hour window of time. This means you are fasting for 14 hours a day. A great start.
- Then move to one day a week of a 24-hour fast. This means you simply skip one breakfast a week. If you are already PK, autophagy cuts in at 16 hours.
- Do a two-day fast once a month. This means you skip two breakfasts and one evening meal.

If you are fighting an acute infection of other condition, put Groundhog Acute (page 149) in place and fast until recovered – this is therapeutic and restful.

If you have underactive thyroid and/or another chronic condition, put Groundhog Chronic in place, follow the fasting programme above and then adjust the frequency of fasting according to how you feel and how symptoms ares regressing. One of the best predictors of longevity is the amount of food consumed. I am greedy and love food. I reckon fasting gives me the best of both worlds – you can be greedy (without bingeing) on feast days and not be hungry, helpless or hapless on fasting days.

Overview and fine-tuning of the PK diet lifestyle

Table C.4: Summary of the PK diet and lifestyle

Problem	Why?	What to do
Addiction to sugar, fruit, caffeine, alcohol, nicotine, cannabis	Addiction masks appetite and we consume for all the wrong reasons. Addictions disturb sleep quality and quantity Addictions mask symptoms	Use addictions occasionally and in moderation
Most Westerners are carbohydrate addicts	Too much carb drives pathology: fatigue, obesity, type 2 diabetes, cancer, arteriosclerosis and dementia ('type 3 diabetes')	Get into ketosis – use the ketone breath meter to demonstrate such. In ketosis your muscle and liver glycogen sponges are squeezed dry. That means the body can easily deal with any carbs in the diet. (I am usually in ketosis after breakfast, always in ketosis late afternoon)
	If you overwhelm the ability of the upper gut to digest, then it will ferment and that drives even more pathology. Symptoms include gastritis, reflux, GORD, bloating, burping and foggy brain. Pathology includes inflammation, autoimmunity including Hashimoto's, toxicity and much more	Do not overeat carbs. Take vitamin C to bowel tolerance. Lugol's iodine 15% 2-3 drops at night. Fast
Some carbohydrate is fine, just not too much!	Sugars are needed as building blocks (to make DNA, RNA and ATP) and to detox (glucuronidation). The body can make sugar from proteins	Use the ketone breath meter to monitor how you flip in and out of ketosis – that makes sure you are not over-loading with carbs. Get your carbs from vegetables, nuts and seeds. If you never blow positive for ketones, fast until you get a positive test

Table C.4 (cont'd)

Problem	Why?	What to do
We have been led to believe fats are bad for us but they are highly desirable	As fuels – the keto-adapted athlete performs 10-15% better. As building materials – for energy delivery mitochondria, all cells especially those of the brain and immune system	Eat fatty meats, fish, poultry, duck, eggs, butter. Lard, dripping, goose fat, coconut oil are ideal for cooking. Oils must not be heated (or you create toxic trans fats)
Dairy products are meant for young mammals	Too much dairy is a risk for: • Cancer • heart disease • osteoporosis	Cut out all dairy products. The safest dairy products are butter and ghee. Vegan butters, cheeses, coconut milks and coconut yoghurts make superb replacements
Western diets are low in fibre	Fibre makes for chewing which stimulates digestion. It is essential for the friendly fermentation in the large bowel to produce: fuel (short-chain fatty acids), vitamins (B and K) and bulk for effortless passage of stool. Friendly fermentation programmes the immune system and protects against infection	Eat sufficient fibre until you pass a Bristol stool chart number 4, once or twice daily effortlessly, ideally using a squatty potty. Make the PK linseed bread which is 27% fibre, 2% carb (see our book *Paleo-Ketogenic: The Why and The How*)
Processed food is often addictive	High-carb, low-protein. Deficient in micronutrients. Toxic with chemicals. Low in fibre	Do not eat processed food – eat real food
Western diets are lacking in variety	We know that the more diverse the microbes of the gut the healthier. Each microbe has a liking for a certain food	Keep ringing the changes and eat foods that are in season Eat as varied a diet as possible
	Once you have conquered addiction your body and brain will tell you what and how much to eat. It has separate appetites for protein, fat, carb, salt, micronutrients and possibly more	Listen to your appetite – if you fancy it you probably need it

	If we become ill, we develop an appetite for healing herbs, essential oils and other remedies. This is well established in animals and is called 'zoopharmacognosy'[2]	Listen to your appetite, brain and body. When ill, it may tell you to fast and sniff!
Low-calorie dieting	Many people half starve themselves in a misguided attempt to lose weight. This simply makes you tired, cold, foggy brained and depressed	Make sure you are eating sufficient calories. Use the method above to work out your daily need
Vitamin C deficiency is pandemic	Humans have lost the ability to synthesise vitamin C from sugars	Take vitamin C as ascorbic acid little and often through the day. Everyone's dose is different; take it to bowel tolerance or to urine tolerance (test with vitamin C urine test strips* Most need 5-8 g (5000-8000 mg) daily, much more for acute infections
Micronutrient deficiencies are pandemic	Soils are depleted by modern agriculture and lack of recycling of human compost back to the soils	Take a good multivitamin and Sunshine Salt 5 grams daily
Allergies are common	Irritable bowel, headaches, asthma, arthritis are often allergy driven	Cut out common allergens e.g. dairy, gluten, yeast. Cut out known allergens
Low-protein diets are common	Protein is an essential on a daily basis – it cannot be stored. Protein leverage: Too little in the diet will stimulate the appetite to eat any food (often high-carb) until the protein appetite is satisfied; consequent overeating calories causes obesity	Calculate your protein requirement as above
Snacking Food constantly present in the upper gut	This means the stomach never has a chance to heal, repair and restore normal acidity resulting in poor digestion and fermenting upper gut	Eat all food within a 10-hour window of time. Do not snack. Breakfast at 7.30am, light lunch, supper by 5.30. (Early supper improves sleep quality)

*Footnote: Vitamin C urine test strips are readily available online. For example, see this product:
www.amazon.co.uk/Vitamin-Strips-Urine-Analysis-VitaChek-C/dp/B00K2265JQ

Table C.4 (cont'd)

Problem	Why?	What to do
	Fasting has great benefits – primitive man did not eat three meals a day. It: • switches on autophagy which protects against cancer and degeneration • switches on stem cells for new growth and repair • clears the foggy brain • squeezes dry the glycogen sponge and gets you into ketosis rapidly	Do 24-hour fast weekly (e.g. skip breakfast and lunch for one day a week). Do a 48-hour fast monthly
Perhaps do longer fasting once a year		
Low levels of exercise	Do the right sort of daily anaerobic exercise to increase muscle bulk. This keeps you strong and increases your BMR (see *Ecological Medicine* Chapter 23 Exercise – this must be the right sort to afford overall gains)	With more muscle you need to eat more. Jolly good – I love food and I am greedy!

Appendix D

The Groundog regimes

Introduction to the Groundhog regimes
Groundhog Basic
Groundhog Acute
Groundhog Chronic

Because I constantly refer back to the basic approach outlined in this Appendix, which is fundamental to the treatment of all infections, and by inference to the avoidance of the major killers (cancer, heart disease, dementia) which are all now known to be driven by chronic infection, I call them the Groundhogs. In the film *Groundhog Day* the protagonist is caught in a time loop where the same day is repeated again and again until there is a shift in his understanding; my Groundhog regimes represent another sort of loop that bears constant repetition. The point here is that the Groundhogs done well will do much to prevent acute illness developing and chronic disease getting a foothold.

It is also the case that the Groundhogs will change through life as we are exposed to new infections and as our defences decline with age. The key principles are:

- All should do Groundhog Basic all (well, most) of the time.
- All should be prepared to upgrade to Groundhog Acute (page 149) to deal with unexpected and sudden infectious challenges – get that First Aid box stocked up now (page 151)!
- We will all need to move to Groundhog Chronic as we age and acquire an infectious load (page 154).

In summary. we use the Groundhogs like this:

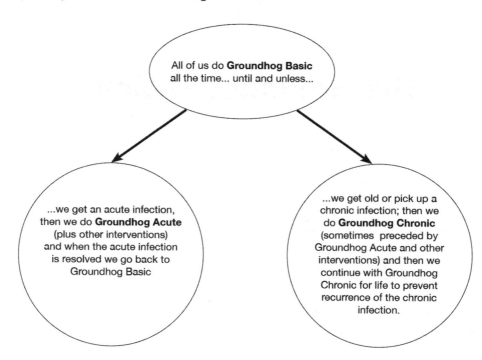

Groundhog Basic

The supplements noted in Table D.1 are what I call the 'basic package' – they are what we should all be doing all the time, especially the kids.

Table D.1: Groundhog Basic

What to do	Notes
The Paleo-Ketogenic diet • high fat, high fibre, very low carb • probiotic foods like kefir and sauerkraut • no dairy or grains • two meals a day with no snacking	See Appendix C and, for more detail, our books *Prevent and Cure Diabetes – delicious diets not dangerous drugs* and *Paleo-Ketogenic: The Why and the How*
A basic package of nutritional supplements – multi-vitamins, multi-minerals and vitamin D	A good multi-vitamin and Sunshine salt 1 tspn daily with food. 1 dsp hemp oil
Vitamin C	Take vitamin C 5 g little and often through the day; I suggest 1 tsp of ascorbic acid in your 1 litre water bottle. (See Appendix E for more detail)
Sleep 8-9 hours between 10:00 pm and 7:00 am	More in winter, less in summer
Exercise at least once a week when you push yourself to your limit	It is anaerobic exercise that produces lactic acid and stimulates the development of new muscle fibres and new mitochondria
Herbs, spices and fungi in cooking	Use your favourite herbs, spices and fungi in cooking and food, and lots of them – Yum yum!
If fatigue is an issue - address energy delivery mechanisms as best as you can	See our book *Diagnosing and Treating Chronic Fatigue Syndrome and Myalgic Encephalitis: its mitochondria not hypochondria*
Heat and light	Keep warm; sunbathe at every opportunity
Use your brain	Foresight: Avoid risky actions like kissing,* unprotected sex. Caution: Avoid vaccinations; travel with care Circumspection: Do not suppress symptoms with drugs; treat breaches of the skin seriously

It is so important to have all the above in place and then at the first sign of any infection take vitamin C to bowel tolerance and use iodine for local infections, because:

- You will feel much better very quickly.
- Your immune system will not be so activated that it cannot turn off subsequently. So many patients I see with ME started their illness with an acute infection from which they never recovered – their immune system stayed switched on.
- The shorter and less severe the acute infection, the smaller the chance of switching on an inappropriate immune reaction, such as autoimmunity. Many viruses are associated with one type or another of arthritis – for example, 'palindromic rheumatism'.[†] I think of this as viral allergy.
- The shorter and less severe the acute infection, the smaller the chance the microbe concerned has of making itself a permanent home in your body. Many diseases, from Crohn's and cancer to polymyalgia and Parkinson's, have an infectious driver (see our book *The Infection Game: Life is an arms race*).

*Oscar Wilde (16 October 1854 – 30 November 1900) knew this, perhaps for different reasons than the risk of infection, when he wrote that: 'A kiss may ruin a human life.' (From *A Woman of No Importance* (is there ever such a thing? asks Craig))

[†]**Note:** Palindromic rheumatism is rheumatism that comes and goes. The word 'palindrome' was coined by English playwright Ben Johnson in the 17th Century from the Greek roots *palin* (πάλιν: 'again') and *dromos* (δρόμος; 'way, direction'). The first known palindrome, written as a graffito, and etched into the walls of a house in Herculaneum, reads thus: *'sator arepo tenet opera rotas'* – 'The sower Arepo leads with his hand the plough'. (idiomatic translation). Much of the graffiti (graffito is the singular of graffiti) found in Pompeii and Herculaneum are somewhat bawdy, some focusing on what the local ladies of the fine houses would like to do with certain named gladiators or, indeed, vice-versa... The authors leave it to the readers to do their own research.

Groundhog Acute – what we should all do at the first sign of any infection, no matter what or where

At the first sign of any infection, you must immediately put in place Groundhog Acute. Do not forget the wise advice of Dr Fred Klenner (BS, MS, MD, FCCP, FAAFP, 1907 – 1984): 'The patient should get large doses of vitamin C in all pathological conditions while the physician ponders the diagnosis.' Strike soon and strike hard because time is of the essence. I repeat myself here because it is so important:

- You will feel much better very quickly.
- Your immune system will not be so activated that it cannot turn off subsequently. So many patients I see with ME started their illness with an acute infection from which they never recovered – their immune system stayed switched on.
- The shorter and less severe the acute infection, the smaller the chance of switching on an inappropriate immune reaction, such as autoimmunity. Many viruses are associated with one type or another of arthritis – for example, 'palindromic rheumatism'[†]. I think of this as viral allergy.
- The shorter and less severe the acute infection, the smaller the chance the microbe concerned has of making itself a permanent home in your body. Many diseases, from Crohn's and cancer to polymyalgia and Parkinson's, have an infectious driver (see page 75 and our book *The Infection Game*).

At the first sign of the tingling, sore throat, runny nose, malaise, headache, cystitis, skin inflammation, insect bite, or whatever… Table D.2 shows what you should do.

Table D.2: Groundhog Acute

What to do	Why and how
The paleo-ketogenic (PK) diet • high fat, high fibre, very low carb • probiotic foods like kefir and sauerkraut • no dairy or grains • two meals a day; no snacking	See Appendix C and, for more detail, our books *Prevent and Cure Diabetes – delicious diets not dangerous drugs* and *Paleo-Ketogenic: The Why and the How*
You may consider a fast – this is essential for any acute gut infection. Drink rehydrating fluids – that is, Sunshine salt 5 g in 1 litre of water ad lib	'Starve a cold; starve a fever' (No, not a typo – starve *any* short-lived infection)
Vitamin C to bowel tolerance. The need for vitamin C increases hugely with any infection. Interestingly our bowel tolerance changes so one needs a much higher dose to get a loose bowel motion during an infection. If you do not have a very loose bowel motion within one hour of taking 10 g, take another 10 g. Keep repeating until you get diarrhoea Most of us need 3-4 doses to abolish symptoms	As explained in greater detail in Appendix E, vitamin C greatly reduces any viral, or indeed any microbial, load in the gut (be aware that some of the infecting load of influenza virus will get stuck onto the sticky mucus which lines the lungs and is coughed up and swallowed) Vitamin C improves the acid bath of the stomach. Vitamin C protects us from the inevitable free-radical damage of an active immune system
A good multi-vitamin Sunshine salt 1 tspn daily in water 1 dsp hemp oil	Sunshine salt in water because you should be fasting at a ratio of 5 g (1 tsp) in 1 l water to provide a 0.5% solution
Take Lugol's iodine 12%: 2 drops in a small glass of water every hour until symptoms resolve. Swill it round your mouth, gargle, sniff and inhale the vapour	It is well documented that 30 seconds of direct contact with iodine kills all microbes
With respiratory symptoms, put 4 drops of Lugol's iodine 12% into a salt pipe and inhale for 2 minutes; do this at least four times a day. Apply a smear of iodine ointment inside the nostrils	As above, 30 seconds of direct contact with iodine kills all microbes This will contact-kill microbes on their way in or on their way out, rendering you less infectious to others
Apply iodine ointment 10% to any bite, skin break or swelling	Again, iodine contact-kills all microbes and is absorbed through the skin to kill invaders

Consume plenty of herbs, spices and fungi	If you are still struggling, then see *The Infection Game – life is an arms race* for effective herbal preparations and how to deal with complications of infection
Rest • listen to your symptoms and abide by them • sleep is even more important with illness	I see so many people who push on through acute illness and risk a slow resolution of their disease with all the complications that accompany such. The immune system needs the energy to fight! I find vitamin C to bowel tolerance combined with a good night's sleep has kept me cold free and flu free for 35 years
Heat • keep warm	Fevers kill all microbes. Some people benefit from sauna-ing. Do not exercise!
Light • sunshine is best	Sunbathe if possible.
Use your brain • do not suppress symptoms with drugs	Symptoms of infection help the body fight infection. Anti-inflammatory drugs inhibit healing and repair – they allow the microbes to make themselves permanently at home in the body
If you develop other acute symptoms…	…see *The Infection Game – life is an arms race* But *all* treatments start with Groundhog Acute

You may consider that doing all the above amounts to over-kill, but when that 'flu or coronavirus epidemic arrives (I originally wrote this text *before* Covid-19 appeared!), as it surely will, you will be very happy to have been prepared and to have these weapons to hand so that you, your family, friends and neighbours will survive. Stock up your Groundhog Acute First Aid box now. As Lord Baden Powell wrote in *Scouting for Boys*, 'Be prepared'; and heed the wisdom of Benjamin Franklin (17 January 1706 - 17 April 1790): 'By failing to prepare, you are preparing to fail.'

The contents of the Groundhog Acute Battle First Aid box

John Churchill, 1st Duke of Blenheim (26 May 1650 – 16 June 1722) was a highly successful General, partly because he made sure his armies were fully equipped for battle. The essence of success is to be prepared with the necessary to combat all assailants. As I have said, strike early and strike hard. Of John Churchill, Captain Robert Parker (who was at the Battle of Blenheim, 13 August 1704) wrote: '…it cannot be said that he ever slipped an opportunity of fighting….' We must be equally belligerent in our own individual battles. Part of this belligerence is preparedness, so keep the following in your own 'Battle First Aid Box' and use it at the first sign of attack.

Table D.3: What to keep in your Battle First Aid box

When	What
For acute infections	
	Vitamin C as ascorbic acid at least 500 g (it is its own preservative so lasts for years) Lugol's iodine 15% - at least 50 ml (it is its own preservative so lasts for years)
Conjunctivitis, indeed, any eye infection	Iodine eye drops e.g. Minims povidine iodine 5% OR 2 drops of Lugol's iodine 15% in 5 ml of water; this does not sting the eyes and is the best killer of all microbes in the eye
Upper airway infections	Lugol's iodine – to be used in steam inhalation, OR Salt pipe into which drizzle 4 drops of Lugol's iodine 15% per dose
Skin breaches	Salt – 2 tsp (10 g) in 500 ml water (approx 1 pint) plus 20 ml Lugol's iodine 15%. Use ad lib to wash the wound. Once clean, allow to dry and then smother with iodine oil (coconut oil 100 ml with 10 ml of Lugol's iodine 15% mixed in) Plaster or micropore to protect
Fractures	If the skin broken – as for Skin breaches above Immobilise If the limb is fractured, wrap in cotton wool to protect and bandage abundantly with vet wrap to splint it Next stop… casualty
Burns	As for skin breaches above If a large burn, then use cling film to protect once cleaned (put the iodine ointment on the cling film first, then apply to the burn) Protect as per fracture above. For a very large burn… next stop casualty

All injuries involving skin breaches	Sterile dressings: Melolin is a good all-rounder Large roll of cotton wool Crepe bandages (various sizes) Micropore tape to protect any damaged area from further trauma Vet wrap bandage – this is wonderful stuff, especially if you are in the wilds, to hold it all together
Gastroenteritis	Sunshine salt: To make up a perfect rehydration drink mix 5 g(1 tsp) in 1 litre of water to give a 0.5% solution
Urine infections	Multistix to test urine D mannose and potassium citrate‡
Bacterial infections	Consider acquiring antibiotics for intelligent use. These should not be necessary if you stick to Groundhog Basic and apply Groundhog Acute BUT I too live in the real world and am no paragon of virtue, so, if you slip off the band wagon:
Dental	Amoxil 500 mg x 21 capsules
ENT and respiratory	Cephalexin 500 mg three times daily
Diverticulitis	Doxycycline 100 mg twice daily (DO NOT USE IN PREGNANCY OR FOR CHILDREN)
Urinary	Trimethoprim 200 g twice daily
Any	If you are susceptible to a particular infection, then make sure you always hold the relevant antibiotic; the sooner you treat, the less the damage, but always start with Groundhog Acute

Putting together such a Battle First Aid Box is as much an intellectual exercise as a practical one and this book, along with our books *The Infection Game – life is an arms race* and *Paleo-Ketogenic – the Why and the How* give such intellectual imperative. As Shakespeare writes in *Henry V*: 'All things are ready, if our mind be so.'

---

‡ Mannose and potassium citrate doses:

D-mannose – One typical product is https://uk.iherb.com/prNow-Foods-D-Mannose-500-mg-120-Veggie-Caps.525. Take 3 x 500 mg capsules one to three times a day

Potassium citrate – These are all example products with their respective doses:

• Effervescent tablets (brand Effercitrate) - take 2 tablets up to three times a day dissolved into a glass of water

• Liquid medicine (brand Cymaclear) - take 2 x 5 ml stirred into a whole glassful of water, up to three times a day

• Sachets (brand Cystopurini) - empty the contents of 1 sachet into a whole glassful of water and stir well before drinking, three times a day.

Groundhog Chronic – what we should all be doing increasingly as we age to live to our full potential

As we age, we acquire infections. My DNA is comprised 15% of retro virus. So is yours. I was inoculated with Salk polio vaccine between 1957 and 1966 so I will probably have simian virus 40, a known carcinogen. I am probably carrying the chickenpox, measles, mumps and rubella viruses because I suffered those as a child. I was also a bit spotty so proprionibacterium acnes may be a potential problem. At least 90% of us have been infected with Epstein Barr virus. I have been bitten by insects and ticks from all over the British Isles so I could also be carrying Lyme (borrelia), bartonella, babesia and perhaps others. I have been a cat owner and could well test positive for bartonella. I have suffered several fractures which have healed but I know within that scar issue will be lurking some microbes – feed them some sugar and they will multiply and give me arthritis. I have had dental abscesses in the past and have one root filling which undoubtably will also harbour microbes. In the past, I have consumed a high carb diet which inevitably results in fermenting gut. On the good side, my puritanical upbringing means I have been free from STDs (thank you Mum!).

All these microbes have the potential to drive nasty diseases such as leukaemia, lymphoma, dementia, Parkinson's, heart disease, auto-immunity, cancer and so on. See *The Infection Game – life is an arms race* for more detail on this. I cannot eliminate them from my body, I have to live with them. I too am part of the Arms Race of the aforementioned book! Of course, this is a race I will (eventually) lose, but I will settle for losing it when I am 120. I am hoping that Groundhog Chronic will handicap my assailants and stack the odds in my favour.

So, as we age and/or we acquire stealth infections (see *The Infection Game – life is an arms race* for this also), we all need Groundhog Chronic (Table D.4). It is an extension of Groundhog Basic. Most will end up doing something between the two according to their health and history. But as you get older you have to work harder to stay well.

Table D.4: Groundhog Chronic

What to do	Why	What I do My patients always ask me what I do. I am no paragon* of virtue, but I may have to become one eventually!
The paleo-ketogenic (PK) diet: • high fat, high fibre, very low carb • probiotic foods like kefir and sauerkraut • no dairy or grains • Two meals a day and no snacking Source the best quality foods you can find and afford – organic is a great start!	See Appendix C and our books *Prevent and Cure Diabetes – delicious diets not dangerous drugs* and *Paleo-Ketogenic – the Why and the How*	Yes. I do the PK diet 95% of the time. Glass of cider at weekends! Other liberties if eating out or socialising. But my friends are all becoming PK adapted too
Eat daily food within a 10 hour window of time…	…so 14 hours a day when your stomach is empty – this keeps the stomach acid and so decreases the chances of microbes invading. Maintains ketosis	Nearly there… breakfast at 8:00 am, supper 6.30 pm
Consider episodic fasting one day a week	This gives the gut a lovely rest and a chance to heal and repair	I do this some weeks. The trouble is I am greedy and love food!
A basic package of nutritional supplements – multi-vitamins, multi-minerals and vitamin D	A good multi-vitamin and Sunshine salt 1 tsp daily with food. 1 dsp hemp oil	Yes
Glutathione 250 mg daily Iodine 25 mg weekly	We live in such a toxic world we are inevitably exposed. Glutathione and iodine are helpful detox molecules (some people do not tolerate iodine in high doses)	Yes

*The English noun 'paragon' comes from the Italian word *paragone*, which is a touchstone – a black stone that is used to tell the quality of gold.

Table D.4 (cont'd)

What to do	Why	What I do My patients always ask me what I do. I am no paragon* of virtue, but I may have to become one eventually!
Vitamin C to 90% of bowel tolerance, including 5 grams last thing at night. Remember this will change with age, diet and circumstance	With age, influenza becomes a major killer. With Groundhog you need never even get it!	Yes. I currently need 8 grams in 24 hours. BUT I never get colds or influenza that last more than 24 hours
Lugol's iodine 15% 2 drops daily in water.	Swill round the mouth and swallow last thing at night	Yes
Make sure your First Aid box is stocked	So, you have all your ammo to hand to hit new symptoms hard and fast	Yes – even when I go away, I take this – often to treat sickly others!
Sleep 8-9 hours between 10:00 pm and 7:00 am Regular power nap in the day Good sleep is as vital as good diet	More in winter, less in summer	Yes
Exercise within limits. By this I mean you should feel fully recovered next day. If well enough, once a week push those limits, so you get your pulse up to 120 beats per min and all your muscles ache. It is never too late to start!	No pain no gain. Muscle loss is part of ageing - exercise slows this right down Helps to physically dislodge microbes from their hiding places. I suspect massage works similarly	Yes. Thankfully I am one of those who can and who enjoys exercise
Take supplements for the raw materials for connective tissue such as glucosamine. Bone broth is the best!	With age we become less good at healing and repair	Yes
Herbs, spices and fungi in cooking	Use your favourite herbs, spices and fungi in cooking and food, and lots of them!	Yes. Because I love food!
Consider herbs to improve the defences – see *The Infection Game – life is an arms race*	Astragalus, cordyceps and rhodiola	Sometimes when in stock and I remember

Address energy delivery mechanisms as below	See our book *Diagnosing and treating Chronic fatigue syndrome and myalgic encephalitis: its mitochondria not hypochondria*	Yes Craig– I've got the book![†]
Take the mitochondrial package of supplements daily vis: Co Q 10 100 g, niacinamide slow release 1500 mg, acetyl L carnitine 500 mg. D ribose 5-10 grams at night if you have really overdone things	With age fatigue becomes an increasing issue because our mitochondrial engines start to slow. The ageing process is determined by mitochondria. Look after them!	Yes I don't take carnitine because I eat meat and my digestion is good
Mitochondria may be going slow because of toxins. Consider tests of toxic load to see if you need to do any detox	A good all-rounder is Genova urine screen with DMSA 15 mg per kg of body weight. You can get this test through https://naturalhealthworldwide.com/	This is the only test I have ever done on myself! It showed background levels of toxic minerals
Check your living space for electromagnetic pollution	You can hire a detection meter from Healthy house www.healthy-house.co.uk/electro/meters-and-monitors	Yes. The cordless phone has gone! I never hold a mobile phone to my ear – I use the speaker Turn wifi off at night
Review any prescription medication – they are all potential toxins! The need for drugs is likely to be symptomatic of failure to apply Groundhog	Ask yourself why you are taking drugs? See our book *Sustainable Medicine*. Once Groundhog is in place many drugs can be stopped. Taking prescription drugs is the fourth commonest cause of death in Westerners	I never take symptom-supressing medication. This has allowed full and now pain-free recovery from three broken necks (horses again) and other fractures

[†]Sarah has commented thus: 'Yes, Craig – I've got the book!' This is a reference to our consultations. Often Sarah is heard to say (in answer to my many questions): 'It's in that book, the one you wrote,' to which I answer: 'Yes, Sarah – I've got the book!'

Table D.4 (cont'd)

What to do	Why	What I do
		My patients always ask me what I do. I am no paragon* of virtue, but I may have to become one eventually!
Consider tests of adrenal and thyroid function, as described in this book, since these glands fatigue with age and chronic infection	See Appendix A Core temperatures are helpful for fine tuning adrenal and thyroid function with glandulars – see page 42	I find glandulars very helpful and currently take thyroid glandular 60 mg in the morning and 30 mg midday Adrenal glandular 500 mg once daily
Heat and light	Always keep warm. Sunbathe at every opportunity. Holidays in warm climates with sunbathing and swimming are excellent for killing infections and detoxing	I am a pyromaniac! My kitchen is lovely and warm with a wood-fired range. I work in my conservatory with natural light. I sunbathe as often as wet Wales permits. Do not forget hyperthermia and light are a good treatment for chronic infections
Use your brain	Foresight: Avoid risky actions like kissing[†], unprotected sex Caution: Avoid vaccinations. Chose travel destinations with care. Circumspection: Do not symptom suppress with drugs, treat breaches of the skin seriously	I have to say that with age this is much less of an issue! No vaccinations. No foreign travel except to the continent to see my daughter and to do lectures

Appendix E

Vitamin C

Vitamin C is an immensely useful tool and in recent years has revolutionised my practice. It is the starting point to treat fermenting gut and all infections, acute and chronic, and therefore any condition involving inflammation. It multitasks to improve detoxing, is an essential antioxidant, and is vital for healing and repair. It kills all microbes (bacteria, viruses and fungi) and is toxic to cancer cells. In healthy people it slows the ageing process; in the acutely and chronically sick, vitamin C to bowel tolerance is part of Groundhog Acute and Chronic (Appendix D). In achieving all this vitamin C is completely non-toxic to human cells. (There is much more detail in our book *The Infection Game: Life is an arms race*.)

Vitamin C was the final tool that allowed me to tell my patients that vaccination is redundant since we have a far more effective, and far safer, tool in vitamin C. With vitamin C we get the best of both worlds. Children can safely experience viral infections without risking complications of such, but receive the vital, alive virus immune programming needed to protect against disease later in life, particularly against cancer. The only vaccination I recommend is tetanus*, but this should be postponed until the child is at risk of stabbing a muck-caked pitchfork through her foot. And yes, I have done that too!

The key to vitamin C is the dose. We simply do not take enough of the stuff. The reason is to be found in Nature – all other animals (except guinea pigs, fruit bats and

*Note from Craig: My 'tetanus moment' was whilst climbing a tree at my Nan's. I was reaching to a bird's nest and fell. A strategically placed rusty nail (holding a swing) ripped down my chest from just under the neck to near the tummy button. If you look carefully, you can still see a scar. It is only the second time I ever saw my Nan cry. We went to the hospital for the vaccination. I was over the moon because I had a scar to show off to my school friends.

dry-nosed primates) can synthesise their own vitamin C. Furthermore, the amount generated is matched to requirements – vitamin C synthesis is hugely ramped up to deal with infection. Goats for example may generate 15 grams a day on demand.[1] We humans have lost this essential biochemical function but instead we have our brains. So we must use them!

Thankfully we have a mechanism to determine the dose we require. This will need to be varied from day to day because the body absorbs what it needs and leaves the excess in the gut. This allows us to adjust the dose according to our guts. Turn this logic on its head – the dose required to achieve bowel tolerance is a reflection of our total infectious load, the extent to which we have a fermenting gut as well as our toxic load and possibly other issues. In other words, our bowel tolerance is a measure of our health.

Lower bowel tolerance   =>   **lower infectious load**
High bowel tolerance   =>   **higher infectious load**

How to take vitamin C to bowel tolerance

Do the PK diet (Appendix C) – vitamin C is much better absorbed in the absence of sugar and starch. There is no point killing microbes with vitamin C if you are feeding them at the same time.

Vitamin C is best taken little and often through the day. Ascorbic acid (AA) is ideal – it is the cheapest and most effective form of vitamin C. If the acid is not tolerated then add magnesium carbonate ($MgCO_3$): two parts AA to one part $MgCO_3$ by weight results in a neutral solution. This also gives you a good dose of magnesium.

Add fizzy water to produce a rather delicious drink. The ascorbic acid helps to sterilise the upper gut and prevents fermentation of food. Any microbes inadvertently consumed with foods are killed. Acid further helps digest proteins and also helps the absorption of essential minerals such as iron and zinc.

Once you are PK and vitamin C adapted you should tolerate ascorbic acid well. The cheapest form is fermented from corn but those who are allergic to corn may not tolerate this at all. Failing that, one can get ascorbic acid from sago palm and/or tapioca (see www.nutriwest.com/products/sago-c-500 and www.amazon.co.uk/Ecological-Formulas-Vitamin-C-1000-Tapioca/dp/B003TVA22A).

Bowel tolerance is defined by that dose that starts to give you gut symptoms. In an acute situation where you need large doses of vitamin C quickly to deal with acute infection, you need 10 grams (g) every hour until you get diarrhoea – see below. In the chronic situation, start with 2 g of vitamin C in your daily bottle of water and drink little and often through the day. Increase at the rate of 1 g every day. Eventually you will get symptoms which may be:

- rumbling tummy: this occurs as microbes in the upper gut are killed, swept downstream and fermented by microbes in the lower gut.
- foul-smelling wind: this occurs as excess vitamin C (i.e. that which is not absorbed or used up in the business of killing upper gut fermenters) gets into the large bowel and kills off the friendlies there which are then fermented by other friendlies to produce offensive farts.

Once you have found the dose that causes these symptoms, drop the dose, normally to around 80-90% of that dose that caused the symptoms, and this will be your personal bowel tolerance dose - that is, it will achieve all the desirable outcomes as listed below.

Adjust the daily dose in the longer term. The idea is to find a dose that kills the grams of unfriendly microbes in the upper gut but does not kill the kilograms of friendly microbes in the lower gut. This will depend on several variables that you will have to work out for yourself a dose that:

- allows you to pass a normally formed daily turd.
- with no smelly farting.
- stops you getting coughs, colds and flu when all around are succumbing.
- reduces, gets rid of or reverses any disease symptoms that you may be suffering from. These may be symptoms of the upper fermenting gut or of chronic infection. As you can see from the Cathcart link below you have to get to 90% of bowel tolerance to reverse the symptoms of any disease process.

At the first hint of any infection, such as a tickle in the throat, runny nose, sneeze, cough, feeling unwell, headache, cystitis (well, you know what from bitter experience…):

- Immediately take 10 g of vitamin C (half this dose for children, according to body weight).
- If this does not produce diarrhoea within one hour take another 10 g.
- If this does not produce diarrhoea within one hour, take another 10 g… and so on.

161

Once you have found the dose that gives you diarrhoea, stop taking vitamin C for that day, and then on subsequent days drop the dose to a level where you do not have diarrhoea or other gastric symptoms. This is normally around 80-90% of the dose that caused diarrhoea. Carry on with this reduced does until the infection clears.

Some people need 200 g to get a result. Whilst this may seem like a huge dose, compare this with sugar: four bars of milk chocolate would provide a similar dose of sugar – and vitamin C is legions safer than sugar!

Some people are appalled at the idea of vitamin C causing diarrhoea. Remember this has the additional benefit of flushing out infectious microbes in the gut and reducing the infectious loading dose. I have to say I would rather have a jolly good bowel-emptying crap than suffer the miserable symptoms of flu or a cold for the next two weeks. Indeed, I have not suffered such for 35 years thanks to vitamin C. My father used to say: 'You can't beat a good shit, shave and shampoo.'

Adjust the frequency and timing of subsequent doses to maintain wellness. Remember, the dose is critical. You cannot overdose, you can only under-dose. Just do it!

Research supporting my vitamin C advice

Dr Robert Cathcart

I am not alone in this advice. Dr Cathcart was a similar advocate of high-dose vitamin C. Some helpful clinical details can be seen at: http://vitamincfoundation.org/www.orthomed.com/titrate.htm[2]

Key points of this Vitamin C Foundation paper are:

- Everyone's bowel tolerance dose is unique to them. It will vary through time with age, diet and infectious load. You have to work it out yourself and it will not remain constant.
- You must get to 80% of your bowel tolerance dose for vitamin C to relieve symptoms. This is another useful clinical tool as you can feel so much better so very quickly if you use vitamin C properly.

Cathcart details many diseases that are improved with vitamin C. Interestingly this includes many cases of arthritis. I suspect this illustrates one mechanism of arthritis which is that it is often driven by allergy to gut microbes. Correct this and the arthritis goes. For example, we know ankylosing spondylitis is an inflammation driven by *Klebsiella* in the gut and rheumatoid arthritis is driven by *Proteus mirabilis*.

Dr Paul Marik

From the Eastern Virginia Medical School in Norfolk, Virginia, USA, Marik added intravenous vitamin C to his normal antibiotic protocol for treating patients diagnosed with advanced sepsis and septic shock in his intensive care unit. Before using vitamin C, the mortality was 40%. Mortality is now less than 1%. Had this been a novel antibiotic it would have made headline news.

Dr Marik offered the following observations:

> *In the doses used, vitamin C is absolutely safe. No complications, side effects or precautions. Patients with cancer have safely been given doses up to 150 grams – one hundred times the dose we give. In the patients with renal impairment we have measured the oxalate levels; these have all been in the safe range. Every single patient who received the protocol had an improvement in renal function.*[3]

(Please note anyone receiving *intravenous* vitamin C must be first checked for glucose-6-phosphate dehydrogenase deficiency. High-dose vitamin C in these people may cause a haemolytic anaemia. I can find no evidence of this being an issue for oral vitamin C.)

There is lots more good science and practical detail at 'Ascorbate Web'.[4] And if nothing else, please do remember that vitamin C is Spanish for 'vitamin yes'!

Appendix F

Detoxing

How to get rid of:
- toxic metals
- pesticides
- VOCs and
- mycotoxins

Step 1 in getting rid of these nasties is Groundhog Basic (Appendix D) – diet, supplements, sleep, exercise, sunshine, love. Indeed yes - Groundhog multi-tasks.

Good nutrition is highly protective against toxic stress. Look at thalidomide. This drug was prescribed to women in pregnancy as a 'pregnancy-safe hypnotic' to improve sleep but caused serious birth defects if taken during early pregnancy. This drug was tested in rats, none of whose offspring was abnormal. This was a mystery to researchers, until someone had the bright idea of putting the rats onto nutritionally depleted diets. When this was done, the baby rats developed the foetal abnormality of phocomelia (horribly dubbed 'flipper limbs').[1] It was a combination of toxic stress (the drug) *and* nutritional deficiency (riboflavin – vitamin B2) at a critical stage of foetal development which caused the problem to become apparent. My mother was prescribed thalidomide throughout all four pregnancies, but we all survived unscathed. Thank goodness she was a great cook.

How to reduce to the body's load of VOCs and pesticides using heating regimes

The liver cannot access VOCs (volatile organic chemicals) and pesticides to detox them because they are stuck elsewhere in the body to do as little damage as possible. The places where they end up stuck are the fat tissues and fatty organs (brain and immune system, viz bone marrow and lymph nodes). This is where heating regimes are so helpful – they mobilise chemicals from these tissues.

Many of the pesticides and VOCs are stored in fat, much of which is subcutaneous. The idea of heating regimes is to heat up this subcutaneous fat and literally boil off the toxins. They migrate through the skin onto the surface where they dissolve in the fatty lipid layer that covers the skin. It is not essential to sweat for these regimes to be effective – the idea is to 'boil off' toxins in the subcutaneous layer of skin onto the lipid layer on the surface from where they can be washed off. The washing off is as important as the heat, or toxins will simply be reabsorbed.

Some toxins will mobilise into the bloodstream and that may cause acute poisoning. It is therefore important to start regimes with low heats and short times and build up slowly.

I have now collected data from over 30 patients who have undergone tests of toxicity both before and after these heating regimes. The tests have been chosen for particular situations but include fat biopsies, translocator protein studies and DNA adducts. The tests have proved to my satisfaction that heating regimes are effective. These heating regimes include sauna (traditional and far infrared (FIR)) and Epsom-salts hot baths. I would expect sun-bathing and exercise to be just as effective. Indeed, similar research was conducted by Dr William Rea in America and he used similar regimes of massage, gentle exercise, sauna-ing and showering to achieve very similar biochemical results. He concluded that 63% of patients decreased their levels of toxic chemicals via these regimes of massage and heating.[2]

My experience, roughly speaking, is that 50 episodes will halve the body load. One would expect chemicals to come out exponentially, so one never gets to zero but can end up in some sort of equilibrium with the environment, which is as low as reasonably possible. Indeed, because we live in such a toxic world, I think we should all be doing some sort of heating regime at least once a week. I am lucky enough to be able to exercise; I deliberately overdress to make sure I get hot and sweaty, then shower off subsequently – what a treat that is!

Indeed, it is my view that because we live in such a toxic world we should not wait until we become ill; we should be using detox regimes on a regular basis and those regimes, in my opinion, should include heating regimes. Take advantage of what is available locally to detox your system on a weekly basis. For those people lucky enough to live in a hot climate, an hour of sunbathing followed by a dip in the sea is ideal. We British relish hot baths, and the effect of detoxification is further enhanced by adding Epsom salts into the water. The idea here is that not only are the toxins pulled out by the heat but magnesium and sulphate pass through the skin into the body, both of which are essential co-factors to allow detoxification. This was established in a lovely study by Dr Rosemary Waring who showed that both magnesium and sulphate levels in the blood increased markedly following such hot baths, as did the excretion of magnesium sulphate in the urine. Her formula was for 500 grams of Epsom salts in 15 gallons of water. (We British also love to mix our metric and imperial measurements! OK, OK… 15 gallons is 68 litres.)[3]

For countries with a tradition of such, sauna-ing is an excellent method of detoxifying through the skin. Indeed, I recall a case of one family who were all poisoned by organophosphate and had high levels in their fat biopsies. They decided to take themselves off for a three-week holiday in Eastern Europe at a lovely hotel which offered regular massage, sauna-ing, hot springs and mineral bath treatments. They all cycled from one treatment to the next. The results were little short of astonishing – after three weeks of treatment their toxic load of organophosphates had reduced substantially, almost to background levels.

Some people feel terrible following heating regimes, probably because of die-off reactions (see Appendix G next). It may be that such reactions are a useful clinical measure of one's combined toxic and infectious load. Should they occur, reduce the time, heat and frequency to whatever is bearable. With time, this will improve.

How to reduce the body's load of toxic metals using detox tools

There are many ways to skin a cat, as the saying goes. All the below are of proven effectiveness. Oral chelation gets the quickest results, but some people do not tolerate this well. In practice, I suggest putting in place as many of the tools below as are tolerable and affordable.

Use a chelating agent such as DMSA

The word chelation comes from the Greek, χηλή, *chela*, or a 'crab's claw'. DMSA literally grabs toxic metals so that they can be excreted in urine. Indeed, this is the basis of the urine test for toxic minerals. Because DMSA also chelates friendly minerals, it should be taken only once a week and one should take no friendly minerals on one's 'DMSA day', but then take good doses to rescue the situation for the other six days of the week. My experience is that most poisoned patients need at least 12 weeks of DMSA, after which the test can be repeated. This gives us two points on the graph and an idea of how much more, if any, chelation is required to reduce the body load to an acceptable level. As I have said, one can never get the body load to zero – all one can do is establish a reasonable equilibrium with the external environment.

Table F.1: Supplements which help detox over and above Groundhog Basic

Supplement	Mechanism	Maximum dose
Zinc, selenium and magnesium	Displace toxic metals from binding sites in the body…	Zinc 50 mg Selenium 500 mcg Magnesium 300 mg - no oral maximum dose but diarrhoea if too much
Glutathione	…so the toxic metals can be picked up by glutathione and excreted	No maximum dose but 250-500 mg is usual
Vitamin C to bowel tolerance (see Appendix E)	Vital antioxidant – the final repository of free radicals	The dose is key and everyone is different
	Binds to toxic metals so they can be excreted in urine	Vitamin C also pulls out friendly minerals so it is vital to take sunshine salt to replace the 'lost' 'good' minerals
Iodine	Binds to toxic metals so they can be excreted in urine	Lugol's Iodine 15% 2-4 drops daily
High-fat diet with several dessert-spoons of organic hemp oil	'Washes out' the polluted fats in the body and replaces with clean. Phospholipids can be given intravenously to good effect	Oral fats and oils probably work as well as when given intravenously but the process takes much longer

Vitamin B12 and ensuing correction of homocysteine	Improves the methylation cycle - sticking a methyl group onto toxins renders them water-soluble so they can be peed out	B12 is extremely safe – take at least 5 mg sublingually daily. Consider B12 injections
	If homocysteine low then correct with…	…Methyl B12 as above, methyl B6 (pyridoxal 5 phosphate) 50 mg and methyltetrahydrofolate 800 mcg daily
Adsorbent clays	See below	

Whichever technique is used, retest to make sure it is working. If not, consider the possibility that there is unrecognised ongoing exposure. For example, is the mercury coming from incomplete amalgam removal? Or fish in the diet?

How to reduce the load of mycotoxins

First you need to identify the source of production, which may be outside the body or inside. The main source outside is water-damaged buildings.

From within the body think either:

- fungi fermenting in the gut (see page 187), and/or
- fungi in the airways (see page 76).

Then use clays to mop up mycotoxins from the gut.

Adsorbant clays to get rid of toxic metals and mycotoxins

Many fat-soluble toxins, such as VOCs and pesticides, are excreted in the fatty bile salts, only to be reabsorbed lower down in the intestine. This is called the 'enterohepatic circulation'. However, clays will **ad**sorb (not absorb – yes, I am a pedant) such toxins so they can be excreted in faeces. This is a benign way to remove toxins since they are not mobilised into the bloodstream and so do not cause detox reactions.

Clays will also remove friendly minerals. Thus, I suggest taking them away from food and supplements – for example, last thing at night. There are many clays with good potential, but I tend to use zeolite 3-10 grams stirred into water and swallowed. As a guide, 3 grams is about a heaped teaspoonful. It does not taste too bad – elephants seek out and love river clay* and I am very happy to be compared to an elephant.

Improve energy-delivery mechanisms

All the above functions are greatly demanding of energy. The liver uses 27% of all the energy generated by the body and much of this is consumed by detox enzymes. The kidneys demand constant energy delivery; they do not tolerate anything less. So, for example, a patient who becomes acutely ill with very low blood pressure may damage their kidneys irreparably with kidney failure.

The gut too requires energy to function – indeed, in its ability to absorb essential nutrients and reject the rest, the gut, biochemically speaking, is comparable to a giant nephron.[†]

---

*__Historical note__ – Geophagia is the word used to describe the deliberate consumption of earth, soil or clay. It has been widely regarded as a psychiatric illness. Indeed, the standard reference guide for psychiatrists — the fourth edition of the *Diagnostic and Statistical Manual for Mental Disorders (DSM-IV)* — classifies geophagia as a subtype of 'pica', an eating disorder in which people consume things that are not food, such as cigarette ash. But studies of animals and human cultures suggest that geophagia is not necessarily a madness. The behaviour is prevalent in more than 200 species of animal, including parrots, deer, elephants, bats, rabbits, baboons, gorillas and chimpanzees. It is also well documented in humans, with Pliny (Gaius Plinius Secundus, 23 – 79 AD) describing the popularity of *alica*, a porridge-like cereal that contained red clay as: 'Used as a drug it has a soothing effect... as a remedy for ulcers in the humid part of the body such as the mouth or anus.'[4] Maybe this is another example of the Ancients not knowing why this practice worked but forging ahead anyway, on the strength of the clinical results.

[†]__Linguistic note__: The nephron (from the Greek νεφρός – nephros, meaning 'kidney') is the functional unit of the kidney.

Appendix G

Diet, detox and die-off (DDD) reactions

- Expect to get worse
- See this as a good sign
- Why this happens
- What to do about it.

'The darkest hour is before dawn'

Old English Proverb now universally used*

Expect to get worse before you improve. This may be demoralising but it depends how you see it… and I am an optimist so I see progress in the right direction. Such reactions are a well-recognised phenomenon and are given comforting names such as a 'healing crisis'. Symptoms can be very severe. Often when patients are so ill, they cannot afford to become any worse. I have great sympathy but no easy answers. Understanding the mechanisms may help. You must be a patient patient.

***Footnote:** The English theologian and historian, Thomas Fuller (19 June 1608 – 16 August 1661), is perhaps the first person to commit this phrase to the printed word. His religious travelogue, *A Pisgah-Sight Of Palestine And The Confines Thereof*, 1650, contains this sentence: 'It is always darkest just before the Day dawneth.' Meant metaphorically, this phrase is not 'actually' true although it can be said that it is coldest before dawn. (Please see https://davidson.weizmann.ac.il/en/online/askexpert/sky-darkest-just-dawn for more detail on this[1]) Sometimes, just before sunrise, the sun casts a shadow of the earth into the visible sky and this gives an impression of a sweep of darkness, much akin to that experienced in a total solar eclipse. It could be that this sweep of darkness gave a 'physical' truth to this phrase and led to its common use.

Also expect a bumpy ride – die-off reactions do not follow a smooth course. Be prepared for something like this:

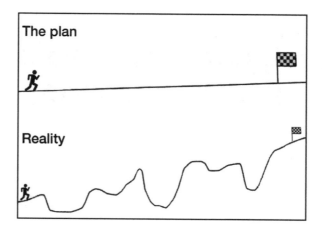

We are fighting a war, but this is composed of many battles. Battles are fought by the macrophage foot soldiers and the lymphocyte officers of our immune system. They can be activated by infections, allergies and toxins. The army throws its all at the invaders and kills them with cytokine bullets. The inflammatory friendly fire that results makes us feel ill. Then the immune armies rest and recover (we feel a bit better) before attacking again – I told you it was a bumpy ride! Then the immune system sweeps up the mess – the parts of dead microbes look like the parts of live ones and this explains 'Herx' reactions (see below).

Diet reactions – there are three common players

1. The metabolic hinterland

The transition from burning carbs to burning fat is difficult and takes time – usually one or two weeks. The body has been used to running on carbs and there is an inertia in the system – it is as if it takes time to 'learn' to burn fat. During this window of time the body cannot get fuel from carbs (because they have been cut out of the diet) so it uses adrenalin to burn fat. To the patient this gives some of the symptoms of low blood sugar because adrenalin is partly responsible for such. We call this 'keto flu', but it is also given the dreadful and confusing name of 'ketogenic hypoglycaemia'. It was first described in the 1960s in children treated for epilepsy with a ketogenic diet. Let me explain further.

We experience the collective symptoms of low blood sugar not only for reasons of low blood sugar, but also for the hormonal response to such:

- fatigue, foggy brain and (indeed for some, especially diabetics on medication) loss of consciousness due to poor energy delivery caused by low blood sugar
- feeling 'hyper', shaky, anxious, possibly with palpitations and fast heart rate, due to adrenalin release
- feelings of hunger and the need to eat, due to gut hormones.

If all is well with the metabolism, the body switches into fat-burning mode (as I've said, it takes one to two weeks for this to happen) and all the above symptoms, which we associate with low blood sugar, disappear. If all is not well with the metabolism, then these symptoms do not disappear and the clinical picture which results is called 'ketogenic hypoglycaemia'. I suspect two causes: lack of carnitine (easily corrected with 1 gram daily) and, more commonly, lack of sufficient thyroid hormone to burn fat, which brings us full circle to the start of this book. That clinical picture is characterised by:

- normal or (even better) low and stable blood sugar levels
- ketosis (confirmed by blood and urine tests)
- the body is burning fat to produce ketones, but it does not have sufficient thyroid hormone to do so efficiently – it relies on extra adrenalin to fat burn
- BUT the adrenalin release gives us nasty symptoms of being 'hyper', shaky, anxious, possibly with palpitations and fast heart rate
- AND STILL gut hormone release – which 'follow' adrenalin release – that is, feelings of hunger and the need to eat
- Clinically, this feels like hypoglycaemia.

Analyse your symptoms. We know keto-adapted athletes improve their performance and the foggy brain clears... despite perhaps feeling dreadful in other respects.

To treat ketogenic hypoglycaemia I recommend: acetyl L carnitine 1 gram daily, and sort out the thyroid problem using this book. But we have to go gently here. In the short term, thyroid and adrenal hormones have very similar actions – that is, to speed things up. If one is still in the metabolic hinterland you may still be spiking adrenalin as your body has yet to 'learn' to use thyroid to burn fat. If you add thyroid hormones to this mix you will end up with the combined effects of thyroid hormones and adrenalin and feel constantly 'hyper'.

2. Addiction reactions

We use addiction to mask unpleasant symptoms such as fatigue, foggy brain and/or pain. Stop the addiction and those symptoms return – ghastly in the short term, great in the long. Obviously sugar and starch addiction are illustrated by the metabolic hinterland[†] but chocolate, caffeine, alcohol, nicotine, cola and other such all have the potential to cause 'train spotting' pain.

3. Allergy reactions

Allergy and addiction seem to be two sides of the same coin. I once had a patient who, even before I was allowed to introduce myself, declared that when he died, he would like to take a cow to heaven with him to ensure a supply of his favourite food. The diagnosis was not difficult. I am not sure of the mechanism by which allergy has this addictive effect, but it is very real.

Detoxification reactions

In the short term, the body can deal with a spike of some toxins by stuffing these into fat and thereby out of harms way. When I do fat biopsies, results come back in milligrams per kilogram. By contrast, blood results come back in micrograms per kilogram. This alone tells us toxic levels in fat are a thousand-fold higher than in blood. Losing weight, heating fat or perhaps even physical massage may mobilise these toxins into the bloodstream and cause an acute poisoning. These toxins, especially pesticides and volatile organic compounds (VOCs), 'boil off' through the skin with heating regimes and cause

---

[†]**Independent film note by Craig**: One of my favourite films is *Hinterland* (not to be confused with the BBC series of the same name). This film is an independent British feature, written and directed by Harry Macqueen. You can sometimes find it here: www.amazon.co.uk/Hinterland-Harry-Macqueen/dp/B00VA61A34. It is the story of an old friendship rekindled, and of self-discovery and heartbreak. Yes, I know – I am such a soppy git! Craig

rashes as the skin reacts allergically to them passing through. The commonest include urticaria and acne-like rashes. The clue can be found in the skin reaction to organo-chlorine poisoning, so called 'chloracne'. I have seen several patients who have been chemically poisoned develop acne whilst detoxing with heat treatments (such as sauna-ing), persist with treatment regardless and eventually find their acne reaction resolved. I can explain this only by a reaction to toxins as they are excreted through the skin.

Some patients being treated with vitamin B12 by injection and/or iodine also get an acne reaction. Both B12 and iodine are good at mobilising toxins from the body. Again, this resolves with time if the sufferer is prepared to put up with the acne in the short term.

Heavy metals stick to proteins and bioconcentrate in organs, particularly the brain, heart, kidneys and bone. They can be mobilised by techniques described in Appendix F: Detoxing, and this too may result in detox reactions.

Mobilising such chemicals is akin to throwing a handful of sand into a finely tuned engine; this may produce almost any symptom. In the very short term, energy delivery mechanism will be impaired. Many toxic metals and chemicals are immuno-toxic – that is, they switch on inflammation.

Die-off reactions ('Herx' or 'Herxheimer')

Die-off reactions were first described by two immunologists, Drs Jarisch and Herxheimer, in patients with syphilis treated with antimicrobials. These symptoms are partly due to endotoxin-like products released by the death of micro-organisms within the body and partly by immune activation. (I think of this as 'allergy to dead microbes', which may explain why Herx reactions are not universal.) Such reactions are potentially very serious and must always be taken as such by at least reducing the dose of any antimicrobial employed and relaxing the regimes that may have triggered the reactions. In the treatment of chronic infection with antimicrobials, I suggest starting with a tiny dose and building up slowly over a few days.

Symptoms of diet, detox and die-off

In practice I have found one can experience:
- Inflammation:
  - systemic symptoms (fever, malaise, aches and pains, depression and fatigue) or local symptoms (acute cold, cough, catarrh, diarrhoea, cystitis etc).
  - local symptoms: it seems to be characteristic of sniffing with an iodine salt pipe that there is an initial increase in mucus and catarrh production; I suspect that as the iodine kills the microbes the body recognises them as invaders and sweeps them out with snot.
- Fatigue: when the immune system is active it takes all our energy, so there is none available to spend physically.
- Foggy brain: the inflamed body is paralleled by the inflamed brain and symptoms of poor energy delivery to the brain result, in particular, with foggy brain, depression and malaise.
- Sickness behaviour: 'Leave me alone. I just wanna go to bed!' This is an energy-saving strategy.

Table G.1: Summary: Getting worse with Groundhog regimes when they should be making you better

Problem	Mechanisms	Action
Metabolic hinterland with ketogenic hypoglycaemia...	Adrenalin is high	Stick with the PK diet. Do not cheat (many do without realising it) or you will never exit the metabolic hinterland. Wait two weeks
...if this persists	Hypothyroidism	Sort out your thyroid using this book! T3 is the fat burner
	Lack of carnitine	You need acetyl L carnitine to burn fat. I suggest 2 grams daily for two months, then a maintenance dose of 500 mg daily (but with a good PK diet, this should not be necessary in the long term)

	'Glycogen storage disorder'[‡]	This may be associated with poor adrenal function – work out the cause. Other than testing for poor adrenal function via an Adrenal Stress Profile Saliva Test (available from Medichecks via www.naturalhealthworldwide.com) further investigations, including blood tests to check blood glucose levels, abdominal ultrasound to look for enlarged liver, or tissue biopsies to directly measure the level of glycogen enzymes may be necessary
Detox reactions	Acute poisoning as chemicals are mobilised from fat	Heating regimes bring toxins out through the skin and this reduces the poisoning effect. Consider zeolite clays which adsorb (not absorb) fat soluble toxins in bile to pull them out in faeces
Addiction withdrawal symptoms in response to withdrawal of social, recreational (this really is a misnomer) and/or prescription drugs	Addiction masks unpleasant symptoms	If too awful then take a tiny dose of your addiction and wean yourself off slowly. Confession time – I love caffeine; consumption waxes and wanes, with detox windows when I avoid it completely[§]
Allergen withdrawal, typically grains or dairy	Do not know for sure – many possibilities	Stick with the PK diet
Symptoms as micronutrient status improves	Mobilising and excreting toxic metals	Consider zeolite clays which adsorb (not absorb) fat-soluble metals in bile to pull them out in faeces

[‡]**Footnote:** GSD is a metabolic disorder caused by enzyme deficiencies. It can affect glycogen synthesis, glycogen breakdown or glycolysis – glucose breakdown – and it typically occurs with muscle and/or liver cells. It can be genetic or acquired.

[§]**Footnote:** regarding caffeine from Craig – Sarah is not alone in her love of caffeine. I drink green tea every day and I make a cup of coffee for my wife, Penny, first thing in the morning every day too. Figures show that 89% of Americans consume some caffeine every day of their lives.[2] According to new research, humans have been drinking caffeinated beverages since at least 750 AD.[3]

Table G.1 (cont'd)

Problem	Mechanisms	Action
Symptoms from heating regimes and/or weight loss	Mobilising pesticides and VOCs from fat	Difficult – slow the regimes down to a point that is bearable
Symptoms from reducing microbial loads with Groundhog Acute or antimicrobial drugs	Herx reactions	Relax the regime and then once tolerated, get up to speed again
Adrenalin spiking with high blood sugar, blood pressure and/or loss of sleep	Any one of the above is a stress and the body responds with adrenalin	Stick with it and hang on to your hat![1]
Skin rashes: urticaria, itching, acne	'allergic' reactions to toxins coming through the skin	Stick with it! It will pass and as it does so other symptoms will improve

All the above illustrates the point that time is a vital part of the diagnostic and therapeutic process. I expect patients to get to this stage after an initial consultation with me that usually concludes with me saying, 'You may love me now, but in a week's time you will hate me'. It is no consolation to tell them that I too have been on the same journey and been equally grumpy about the whole proces. I am sure Craig has experienced the same. (Craig: Indeed, I have but I have never 'hated' Sarah! When going through these DDD reactions, I always have Penny on hand to remind me, 'This is just what Sarah said might happen!')

[1]**Footnote:**: This expression may derive from the need to do just this on rollercoaster rides,- according to lexicographer Eric Partridge (Colloquial; first half of 1900s). This rather suits our 'Reality' graphic above if we can include it. Eric Honeywood Partridge (6 February 1894 – 1 June 1979) was a New Zealand–British lexicographer of the English language, particularly of its slang.

Glossary

Adrenal gland problems

The adrenal gland is the 'gear box' of our car responsible for matching energy demand with energy delivery. It is additionally responsible for controlling the amount of inflammation in the body. It achieves this by secreting adrenaline (the short-term response, measured in seconds and minutes), followed by cortisol (a medium-term response measured in minutes and hours), followed by DHEA (dehydroepiandrosterone – a longer-term stress hormone).

The Hungarian physiologist Hans Selye showed that if you stressed rats, their adrenal glands enlarged to produce more stress hormones (including cortisol and DHEA) to allow the rat to cope with that stress. If the rat had a break and a rest, then the adrenal gland would return to its normal size and recover. However, if the rat was stressed without a break or a rest, he would be apparently all right for some time, but then suddenly collapse and die. When Selye looked at the adrenal glands at this point, they were shrivelled up. The glands had become exhausted.

The current Western way of life is for people to push themselves more and more. Many can cope with a great deal of stress, but everybody has their breaking point. The adrenal gland is responsible for the body's hormonal response to this stress. It produces adrenaline, which stimulates the instant stress hormone response ('fight or flight' reaction), and cortisol and DHEA, which create the short- and long-term stress hormone responses respectively. When the gland becomes exhausted, chronic fatigue develops and tests of adrenal function typically show low levels of cortisol and DHEA. DHEA has only recently been studied because it had not been realised that it had any important actions.

All steroid hormone synthesis starts with cholesterol. The first biochemical step takes place in mitochondria where there is a conversion to pregnenolone. The body can then shunt from pregnenolone either into a stress or catabolic mode (to cortisol) or a rebuilding mode (anabolic hormones such as DHEA, testosterone and oestrogen).

179

Adrenaline (epinephrine)

Adrenaline is the instant stress response hormone that drives our fight or flight reaction. This reaction is characterised by intense arousal (sometimes to the point of anxiety or panic), with a faster heart rate, high blood pressure, higher blood sugar level and sometimes even minor tremor. This is the stress hormone which allows us to move up a gear, sometimes perhaps into overdrive, even in order to kill, within a stressful situation. An obvious evolutionary cause of such stress would be to be hunted by a predator. In our modern, safer lives, I suspect that the commonest stress is falling blood sugar levels and this release of adrenaline is a central part of metabolic syndrome.

Allergy

Allergy is the great mimic. In some ways the immune system is not very clever. It can react to things in only one way – that is, with inflammation. Inflammation causes redness, swelling, pain, heat and loss of function. When you look at a diseased area, you can see those signs, but it does not tell you what the cause is. So, for example, looking at an area of inflamed skin you may not be able to tell if it has been infected, sun-burnt or frozen, had acid spilled on it, or is responding allergically, or whatever. Again, seeing a person with hay fever you may not be able to distinguish this from a head cold. Hay fever sufferers may get a fever too.

You can be allergic to anything under the sun, including the sun. For practical purposes, allergies are split up into allergies to foods, chemicals (including drugs) and inhalants (pollens and micro-organisms such as bacteria, mites, etc).

People with undiagnosed food allergy often initially present with symptoms due to inflammation in the gut (irritable bowel syndrome) and inflammation in the brain (mood swings, depression or brain fog in adults, or hyperactivity in children). However, the inflammation can occur anywhere in the body, resulting in asthma, rhinitis, eczema, arthritis and muscle pain, cystitis or vaginitis, or a combination of symptoms.

Antioxidants

What allows us to live and our bodies to function are billions of chemical reactions in the body which occur every second. These are essential to produce energy, which drives all the processes of life such as nervous function, movement, heart function, digestion and so on. If all these enzyme reactions invariably occurred perfectly, there would be no need for an antioxidant system.

However, even our own enzyme systems make mistakes and the process of producing energy in mitochondria is highly active. When mistakes occur, free radicals are produced. Essentially, a free radical is a molecule with an unpaired electron; it is highly reactive and to stabilise its own structure, it will literally stick on to anything. That 'anything' could be a cell membrane, a protein, a fat, a piece of DNA, or whatever. In sticking on to something, it denatures that something so that it has to be replaced. This means having free radicals is extremely damaging to the body and therefore the body has evolved a system to mop up these free radicals before they have a chance to do such damage, and this is called our antioxidant system. There are many substances in the body which act as antioxidants, but the three most important **frontline antioxidants** are:

- **Co-enzyme Q10.** This is the most important antioxidant inside mitochondria and also a vital molecule in oxidative phosphorylation. Co-Q10 deficiency may also cause oxidative phosphorylation to go slow because it is the most important receiver and donor of electrons in oxidative phosphorylation. People with low levels of Co-Q10 have low levels of energy.
- **Superoxide dismutase (SODase)** is the most important super oxide scavenger in muscles (zinc and copper SODase inside cells; manganese SODase inside mitochondria; and zinc and copper SODase outside cells), and
- **Glutathione peroxidase.** This enzyme is dependent on selenium and glutathione, a 3-amino acid polypeptide, and a vital free-radical scavenger in the bloodstream.

These molecules are present in parts of a million and are in the frontline process of absorbing free radicals. They give up their own electrons and, in the process, they neutralise the unpaired electrons in free radicals. This process continues, via complex sets of reactions, along a chain of antioxidants, such as vitamins A and E, before the ultimate electron donor, vitamin C, gives up its electrons in the same way.

Autoimmunity

Autoimmunity occurs when the immune system has made a mistake. The immune system has a difficult job to do, because it has to distinguish between molecules which are dangerous to the body and molecules which are safe. Sometimes it gets its wires crossed and starts making antibodies against molecules which are 'safe'. For some people this results in allergies, which is a useless inflammation against 'safe' foreign molecules. For others this results in autoimmunity, which is a useless inflammation against the body's own molecules. These are acquired problems – we know that because they become much more common with age. It is likely we are seeing more autoimmunity because of Western lifestyles, diets and pollution. Chemicals, especially heavy metals, get stuck onto cells and change their 'appearance' to the immune system and thereby switch on inappropriate reactions.

Brain fog/Foggy brain

What I mean by brain fog is:

- Poor short-term memory.
- Difficulty learning new things.
- Poor mental stamina and concentration – there may be difficulty reading a book or

181

following a film story or following a line of argument.
- Difficulty finding the right word.
- Thinking one word but saying another.

What allows the brain to work quickly and efficiently is its energy supply. If this is impaired in any way, then the brain will go slow. Initially, the symptoms would be of foggy brain, but if symptoms progress, we end up with dementia. We all see this in our everyday life, with the effect of alcohol being the best example. Short-term exposure gives us a deliciously foggy brain – we stop caring, we stop worrying, it alleviates anxiety. However, it also removes our drive to do things, our ability to remember; it impairs judgement and our ability to think clearly. Medium-term exposure results in mood swings and anxiety (only alleviated by more alcohol). Longer-term use could result in severe depression and then dementia – examples include Korsakoff's psychosis and Wernike's encephalopathy.

Carbohydrate

All vegetable material (grains, pulses, vegetables, salads, fruit, berries, nuts and seeds) contain carbohydrates. These are comprised of:
- Simple monosaccharides and disaccharides. (They all taste sweet, and we call them sugars.)
- Polysaccharides. (These are starches, such as from grain flours or potato.)
- Complex polysaccharides (which we call vegetable fibre).

The sugars and starches are easily digested in our gut and are readily absorbed.

Vegetable fibre cannot be digested by human enzymes; it must be fermented by friendly bacteria in the large bowel. It is fermented to form short chain fatty acids, which are a useful fuel for the body, and they do not affect blood sugar levels. This is what makes high-fibre vegetables such desirable foods.

When looking at food labels, take care. When we 'count carbs', we are looking for the Net Carbohydrate figure – that is Total Carbohydrate MINUS Fibre. When reading food labels, one must understand the difference between how things are disclosed in the US and the EU and UK. For example, if an item, in America, contains 5 grams of Total Carbohydrates, out of which 2 grams consist of Dietary Fibre, then the Net Carbohydrate content of this product is 3 grams (5 grams minus 2 grams). In the UK 'Net Carbohydrates' are already calculated within nutritional labels. Sugars and Starches are disclosed as one entity ('Carbohydrate') and dietary fibre is separately labelled as 'Fibre'. Hence there is no need to calculate Net Carbohydrate content for a product that follows EU and UK labelling rules. For example, if an item from an EU country or the UK is said to contain 3 grams of Carbohydrate and 2 grams of Fibre, then the amount of carbohydrates that will affect blood sugar levels is 3 grams. But do always check and be sure!

Chemical poisoning

The diagnosis of chemical poisoning is suspected from a history of exposures resulting in typical clinical syndromes and confirmed by the appropriate medical tests. There is a series of criteria to be fulfilled to make a confident clinical diagnosis of poisoning by chemicals. The criteria are:

1. The subject was fit and well prior to chemical exposures.
2. There is evidence of exposure to the putative chemicals and toxins.
3. The subject initially developed local symptoms which became worse with repeated exposures.
4. With repeated exposures a typical clinical picture emerges characterised by chronic fatigue syndrome, immune disruption (allergies, autoimmunity, susceptibility to infections), accelerated ageing (so the sufferer gets diseases before their time), neurodegeneration, diabetes and cancer.
5. Similar patterns of disease are seen in other people working under similar conditions.
6. There is similar factual evidence from other individuals who have been poisoned, such as the Gulf War veterans, sheep-dip-poisoned farmers and aerotoxic pilots.
7. There is laboratory evidence of poisoning and effects of that poisoning.
8. There are no other possible explanations for this pattern of symptoms.
9. There is a response to treatment with clinical improvements as a result of detoxification and nutritional and immune support.

Co-enzyme Q10

See antioxidants.

Cortisol

Cortisol is a hormone released by the adrenal gland in response to stress. Essentially, adrenaline is the immediate response, cortisol the medium-term response and DHEA the long-term response. Between these three hormones the body can gear up to stress, maintain that stress response for the required duration, and then normality is restored as the levels of these hormones drop back to normal.

Detoxification

As part of normal metabolism, the body produces toxins which have to be eliminated, otherwise they poison the system. Therefore, the body has evolved a mechanism for getting rid of these toxins and the methods that it uses are as follows:

- Antioxidant system – for mopping up free radicals. See Antioxidants.
- The liver – detoxification by oxidation and conjugation (amino acids, sulphur compounds, glucuronide, glutathione, etc) for excretion in urine.
- Fat-soluble toxins can be excreted in the bile. The problem here is that many of these are

recycled because they are reabsorbed in the gut.
- Sweating – many toxins and heavy metals can be lost through the skin.
- Dumping chemicals in hair, nails and skin, which are then shed.

This system has worked perfectly well for thousands of years. Problems now arise because of toxins which we are absorbing from the outside world. This is inevitable since we live in equilibrium with the outside world. The problem is that these toxins (such as alcohol) may overwhelm the system for detoxification, or they may be impossible to break down (e.g. silicone and organochlorines), or they may get stuck in fatty organs and cell membranes and so not be accessible to the liver for detoxification (for example, many volatile organic compounds). We all carry these toxins as a result of living in our polluted world.

We can help our bodies detoxify by:
- eating a PK diet - increasing the fibre content of food and the bacterial numbers in the gut also facilitates detoxification
- taking a basic package of nutritional supplements – see Appendix D
- heating regimes
- improving antioxidant status.

Fats

The word 'fats' has had a bad press and is associated with putting on weight and being generally 'bad for you'. Fats (and also cholesterol) have been associated with heart disease, but this association is not correct. Please do read 'Good and bad fats' below and also our book *Paleo-Ketogenic: The Why and the How* for more information on why this association is false. Saturated fats provide the perfect fuel. Both saturated and unsaturated fats are essential building blocks for all tissues of the body, especially the brain and immune system.

Good fats and bad fats

Broadly speaking our bodies contain and use two types of fat: medium-chain saturated fats and long-chain unsaturated fats. All fats are made up of fatty acids. It is the structure of these building blocks that determines a fat's character and potential usefulness.

The saturated, medium-chain fats include lard, butter, coconut fat and chocolate fat; we use these as fuel to power the body. For the biochemists, in a saturated fat, every carbon atom is 'saturated' either with another carbon or a hydrogen atom. This renders the fat stiff and stable, so, when heated (which shakes things up), it retains its normal shape. These stiff fats are solid at room temperature.

Generally speaking, medium-chain fats contain between eight and 14 carbon atoms, whilst long-chain fats have more than 14 carbon atoms and short-chain fats, fewer than eight. So, for example, approximately 50% of the fat content of coconut fat is made up of lauric acid (see

Figure G.1). Lauric acid has a melting point of 43.8°C and so is solid at room temperature. It has 12 carbon atoms and is therefore a medium-chain fat. In addition, it is saturated. Being a medium-chain saturated fat, it is therefore stiff and stable, retaining its normal shape when heated.

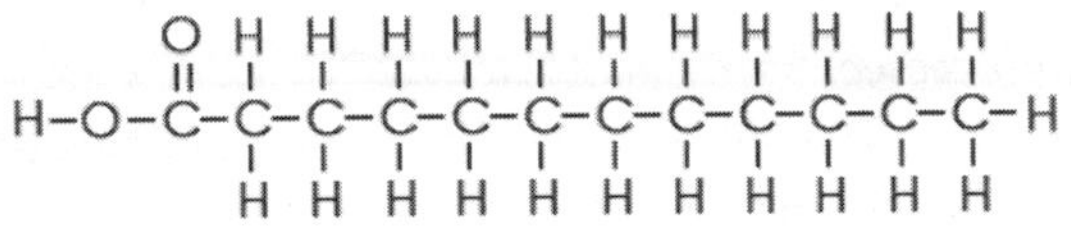

Figure G.1: The structure of a typical saturated fat (lauric acid)

The second type of fat is a long-chain unsaturated fat. The occasional hydrogen atom is 'missing' and so we get a double carbon bond instead. If we have one double carbon bond, then we call this fat 'mono-unsaturated' (such as olive oil) and if we have more than one double carbon bond, we call this fat 'poly-unsaturated' (such as most nut, seed, vegetable and fish oils). This double carbon bond 'kinks' the molecule and the molecule is named according to where it is kinked – such as omega-3, omega-6 or omega-9 depending on where the 'kink' occurs on the carbon chain. Figure G.2 shows how this 'kinking' may look.

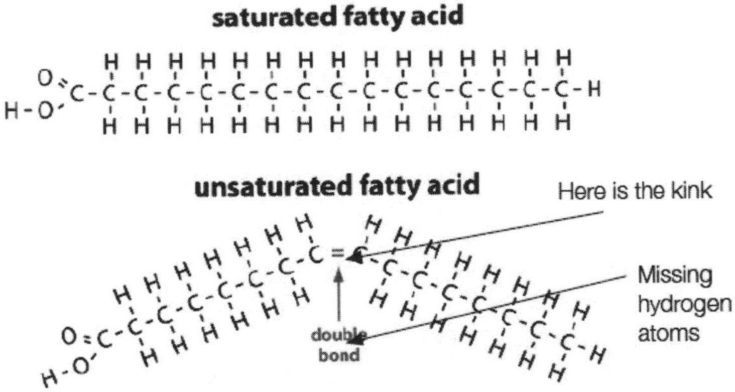

Figure G.2: The structure of a mono-unsaturated fatty acid

These fats are relatively flexible so are liquid at room tempature – we therefore call them 'oils' – and relatively unstable so they can be damaged by heat, for example, more easily than can saturated fats.

We use these fats as building materials – primarily for cell membranes. Indeed, many biological actions, such as energy generation and nerve conduction, take place on such membranes. These fats, or oils, are also called 'essential fatty acids' because the body can't synthesise them for itself; they have to be eaten.

So saturated, mono-unsaturated and polyunsaturated fats can all be good fats. The trouble starts when these good fats are processed.

In Nature, the kinks resulting from the double bonds are all 'left-handed' and are called cis-fats. They fit our biochemistry perfectly. Problems arise when these fats are heated or hydrogenated (processed to render them solid at room temperature) and they flip into a 'right-handed' version; these are called trans-fats. Just as a right hand will not fit into a left handed glove, so trans-fats do not fit our biochemistry, and so they clog up systems and are highly damaging. Figure G.3 shows the problem: the trans-fat is not the same shape as the cis-fat and so will not fit with our biochemistry.

cis-fat molecule

trans-fat molecule

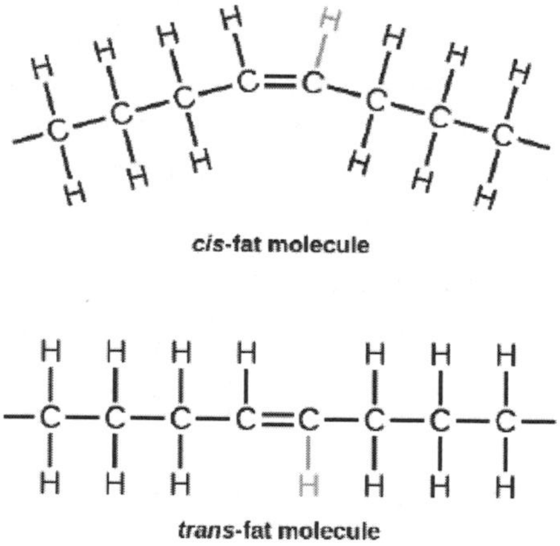

Figure G.3: The crucial difference between a cis-fat and a trans-fat molecule

Because of the consequences of these factors:
- Do not eat hydrogenated fats (as in margarine and 'spreads') – if the fat has been hydrogenated, then the resulting trans-fat will not fit with your biochemistry.
- Cook with saturated fats, such as lard (any animal fat), butter or coconut oil – these fats retain their shape through the cooking process.
- Use cold-pressed oils at room temperature – do not cook with them. Again, the cooking will heat these fats and so 'kinking' may result, meaning that these oils will not fit with our biochemistry.

Normal metabolism is so versatile that the amounts of fat consumed are not critical. General guidelines would be:

Saturated fats: Eat sufficient amounts to maintain weight and energy levels (mental and physical).

Oils: Only tiny amounts of essential fatty acids (EFAs) are required. They are called 'essential' because, like vitamins and minerals, the body cannot synthesise them itself; they have to be consumed. We all need omega-6 (linoleic acid) and omega-3 (alpha linolenic acid) EFAs in the proportion 4:1. These EFAs are present in all oils in varying proportions. I recommend hemp oil because it contains omega-6 and omega-3 in the correct proportion. I suggest a dessert-spoonful daily – it is delicious and can be used in French dressings, mayonnaise or linseed bread (see *Paleo-Ketogenic: The Why and the How* for recipes).

In theory, these parent fats can make all other fatty acids downstream. However, in practice some people cannot do this and additional supplementation with other oils can have great benefit. I additionally recommend a fish oil supplement of 1000 milligrams and evening primrose oil 500 milligrams.

Fermenting gut – 'upper fermenting gut' (see Chapter 3)

The human gut is almost unique amongst mammals: the upper gut is a near-sterile, digesting, carnivorous gut (like a dog's or a cat's) to deal with meat and fat, whilst the lower gut (large bowel or colon) is full of bacteria and is a fermenting, vegetarian gut (like a horse's or cow's) to digest vegetables and fibre. From an evolutionary perspective this has been a highly successful strategy – it allows Inuits to live on fat and protein and other people to survive on pure vegan diets. Problems arose when humans learned to cook and to farm. This allowed them to access new foods – namely, pulses, grains and root vegetables. These need cooking to be digestible. From an evolutionary perspective this has been highly successful and allowed the population of humans to increase at a great rate. However, carbohydrates have the potential to be fermented in the upper gut with problems arising as detailed below.

The stomach, duodenum and small intestine should be almost free from micro-organisms (bacteria, yeasts and parasites – that is, 'microbes'). This is achieved by eating a PK diet, having an acidic stomach which digests protein efficiently and kills the acid-sensitive microbes; then an alkaline duodenum, which kills the alkali-sensitive microbes with bicarbonate; then bile salts (which are also toxic to microbes) and pancreatic enzymes to further digest protein, fats and carbohydrates. The small intestine does more digesting and also absorbs the amino acids, fatty acids, glycerol and simple sugars that result.

Anaerobic bacteria (bacteria that do not use oxygen), largely bacteroides, flourish in the large bowel, where foods that cannot be digested upstream are then fermented to produce many substances that are highly beneficial to the body. Bacteroides ferment soluble fibre to produce short-chain fatty acids – over 500 kcal of energy a day can be generated. This also creates heat to help keep us warm. The human body is made up of 10 trillion cells, yet in our gut we have 100 trillion microbes or more – that is, 10 times as many. Bacteria make up 60% of dry stool weight. There are over 500 different species, but 99% of microbes are from 30–40 species.

In people not eating a PK diet, there are bacteria, yeasts and possibly other parasites existing in the upper gut (stomach, duodenum and small intestine), which means that foods are fermented there instead of being digested. When foods get fermented this can cause symptoms and problems for many reasons such as:

- wind, bloating, heartburn and other digestive problems (so-called irritable bowel syndrome)
- malabsorption
- production of toxins through fermentation or enhanced absorption of toxic metals
- allergy to microbes in the gut (inflammatory bowel disease)
- allergy to microbes at distant sites in the body, manifesting as arthritis, interstitial cystitis, asthma, urticaria, PMR and many others
- in the longer term – cancer, diverticulitis.

Glycogen sponge

All the products resulting from food being digested and then absorbed in the gut pass via the portal vein to the liver. These products are toxic. So, for example, if this toxic load were to pass straight into the systemic bloodstream, we would rapidly lose consciousness and succumb. This occurs in liver failure. One of the toxins in the portal vein is sugar. This is like the petrol in our car – essential for it to run but highly dangerous in large amounts. The liver glycogen sponge prevents the tsunami of sugar in the portal vein from getting into the systemic bloodstream by way of a mopping-up operation. The liver achieves this by rapidly shunting sugar in the blood into the more complex storage form, glycogen, and holding it safely in store, from where it can be used as a pantry when blood sugar levels fall. In this respect the liver has a sponge-like effect. Should sugar levels in the systemic bloodstream fall, then the glycogen sponge can correct this by 'squeezing dry'.

Glycogen can also be stored in the muscles so these too can act as glycogen sponges to be squeezed dry, as needed.

Graves' disease

Graves' disease is an autoimmune condition (see Glossary entry above for 'autoimmune') whereby the immune system mistakenly attacks the thyroid, causing it to become overactive – that is, hyperthyroidism. Graves' disease mostly affects young or middle-aged women and often runs in families. Smoking can also increase your risk of getting it. In addition, other causes that have been identified include viral infections and related vaccines:

- SARS-CoV-2 (COVID) vaccination.[1]
- Epstein Barr virus, also known as 'glandular fever' or 'mononucleosis'. Janegova et al 2015 found that 81% of Hashimoto's thyroiditis cases and 63% of Graves' disease cases had EBV proteins evident in the thyroid gland and therefore proposed an aetiological role of EBV for these autoimmune thyroid diseases.[2]
- Other viruses. Rachel Desailloud and Didier Hober (2009) present epidemiological and virological evidence, along with case reports to support this and conclude: '...evidence of the presence of viruses or their components in the organ... for retroviruses (HFV) and mumps in subacute thyroiditis, for retroviruses (HTLV-1, HFV, HIV and SV40) in Graves' disease and for HTLV-1, enterovirus, rubella, mumps virus, HSV, EBV and parvovirus in Hashimoto's thyroiditis.'[3]

Hashimoto's thyroiditis

Hashimoto's is also known as 'chronic lymphocytic thyroiditis'. It is an autoimmune disease. Autoimmune diseases happen when the body's natural defence system can't tell the difference between own cells and foreign cells, causing the body to mistakenly attack the body's own cells. In Hashimoto's, the thyroid gland is attacked and is gradually destroyed. Complications over time include:

- painless goitre (swelling at the front of the neck)
- hypothyroidism, with all the symptoms associated (see Chapter 1).

Also, over time the thyroid shrinks in size and a further potential complication includes thyroid lymphoma.

Hashimoto's thyroiditis is thought to be caused by a combination of genetic and environmental factors, with family history also being a significant risk, as is having other autoimmune diseases, the so called 'multiple autoimmune syndrome'[4] Diagnosis is confirmed by blood test for TSH and free T4 and especially by the presence of thyroid peroxidase antibodies.[5]

Environmental risk factors include:

- Epstein Barr virus.[6]
- Mould.[5]
- Other viruses.[2]

See also the Glossary entry for Graves' disease.
Treatment is as described in this book.

Hypoglycaemia (see also the mis-named 'Ketogenic hypoglycaemia')

'Hypoglycaemia' is the term used for blood sugar being at too low a level. To explain how this happens it is necessary to describe how sugar levels are controlled.

It is critically important for the body to maintain blood sugar levels within a narrow range. If the blood sugar level falls too low, energy supply to all tissues, particularly the brain, is impaired. However, if blood sugar levels rise too high, then this is very damaging to arteries and the long-term effect of arterial disease is heart disease and strokes. This is caused by sugar sticking to proteins and fats to make AGEs (advanced glycation end-products) which accelerate the ageing process.

Normally, the liver controls blood sugar levels. It can convert glycogen stores inside the liver to release sugar into the bloodstream minute by minute in a carefully regulated way to cope with body demands, which may fluctuate from minute to minute. Excess sugar flooding into the system after a meal can be mopped up by muscles, but only so long as there is space there to act as a sponge. This occurs when we exercise. This system of control works perfectly well until we upset it by eating a high-carb diet and/or not exercising. Eating excessive sugar at one meal, or excessive refined carbohydrate, which is rapidly digested into sugar, can suddenly overwhelm the muscle and the liver's normal control of blood sugar levels.

We evolved over millions of years eating a diet that was very low in sugar and had no refined carbohydrate. Control of blood sugar therefore largely occurred as a result of eating this PK diet and exercising vigorously in the course of daily life, so any excessive sugar in the blood was quickly burned off. Nowadays the situation is different: we eat large amounts of sugar and refined carbohydrate and do not exercise sufficiently to burn off this excess sugar. The body therefore has to cope with this excessive sugar load by other mechanisms.

When food is digested, the sugars and other digestive products go straight from the gut in the portal vein to the liver, where they should all be mopped up by the liver and processed accordingly. If excessive sugar or refined carbohydrate overwhelms the liver, the sugar spills over into the systemic circulation. If not absorbed by muscle glycogen stores, high blood sugar results, which is extremely damaging to arteries. If we were exercising hard, this would be quickly burned off. However, if we are not, then other mechanisms of control are brought into play. The key player here is insulin, a hormone secreted by the pancreas. This is very good at bringing blood sugar levels down and it does so by shunting the sugar into fat. Indeed, this includes the 'bad' cholesterol LDL. There is then a rebound effect and blood sugars may well go too low – in other words, hypoglycaemia occurs. Low blood sugar is also dangerous to the body because the energy supplied to all tissues is impaired.

Subconsciously, people quickly work out that eating more sugar alleviates these symptoms, but of course they invariably overdo things; the blood sugar level then goes high, and they end up on a roller-coaster ride of their blood sugar level going up and down throughout the day.

Ultimately, this leads to 'metabolic syndrome' or 'syndrome X' – a major cause of disability and death in Western societies, since it is the forerunner of diabetes, obesity, cardiovascular disease, degenerative conditions and cancer.

Hypothyroidism – underactive thyroid

An underactive thyroid is a very common cause of fatigue, often as a knock-on effect of a general suppression of the hypothalamic-pituitary-adrenal axis – that is, the coordinated functioning of those three glands. Symptoms of hypothyroidism arise for four reasons – either the gland itself fails (primary thyroid failure), or the pituitary gland which drives the thyroid gland into action under-functions, or there is failure to convert inactive thyroxine (T4) to its active form (T3), or there is thyroid-hormone receptor resistance. In summary, the four types of hypothyroidism are:

- Primary hypothyroidism – when the thyroid is malfunctioning.
- T3 hypothyroidism – when the thyroid cannot convert inactive T4 to the active T3 because of deficiency or blocking.
- Secondary hypothyroidism – when the pituitary gland is malfunctioning.
- Thyroid hormone receptor resistance – when the circulating thyroid hormones are blocked or inhibited, for example by reverse T3 (see page 201) or prescription drugs such as beta blockers.

The symptoms of these three problems are the same, but blood tests show different patterns:

- In **primary thyroid failure**, blood tests show high levels of thyroid stimulating hormone (TSH) and low levels of T4 and T3.
- In **pituitary failure**, blood tests show low levels of TSH, T4 and T3.
- If there is a **conversion problem**, TSH and T4 may be normal, but T3 is low.
- In **thyroid hormone receptor resistance**, there is a high TSH, high T4 and high T3.

There is another problem too, which is that the so-called 'normal range' of T4 is probably set too low. I know this because many patients with low normal T4 often improve substantially when they are started on thyroid supplements to bring levels up to the top end of the normal range.

Inflammation

Inflammation is an essential part of our survival package. From an evolutionary perspective, the biggest killer of Homo sapiens (apart from Homo sapiens) has been infection, with cholera claiming a third of all deaths, ever. The body has to be alert to the possibility of any infection, to all of which it responds with inflammation. However, inflammation is metabolically expensive and inherently destructive. It has to be, in order to kill infections by bacteria, viruses, parasites or whatever. For example, part of the immune defence involves a 'scorched earth' policy – tissue immediately around an area of infection is destroyed so there is nothing for the invader to parasitise.

The mechanism by which the immune system kills these infections is by firing free radicals at them. However, if it fires too many free radicals, then this 'friendly fire' will damage the body itself. Therefore, for inflammation to be effective it must be switched on, targeted, localised and then switched off. This entails extremely complex immune responses; clearly, there is great potential for things to go wrong.

Inflammation is also involved in the healing process. Where there is damage by trauma, there will be dead cells. Inflammation is necessary to clear away these dead cells and lay down new tissues.

Inflammation is characterised by heat and redness (heat alone is antiseptic), combined with swelling, pain and loss of function, which immobilises the area being attacked by the immune system. This is necessary because physical movement will tend to massage the infection to other sites.

If one looks at life from the point of view of the immune system, it has a very difficult balancing act to manage. Too little reaction and we die from infection; too much reaction is metabolically expensive and damaging. If switched on inappropriately, the immune system has the power to kill us within seconds, an example of this being anaphylaxis.

Insulin resistance

Insulin resistance develops as cells in your muscles, fat and liver fail to respond to insulin because they are overwhelmed by sugar from high-carbohydrate diets. This leads to metabolic syndrome (see Glossary entry on page 194) and eventually to diabetes. There is much more detail about these mechanisms of illness in our book *Prevent and Cure Diabetes: Delicious diets not dangerous drugs*. Insulin resistance and diabetes are completely reversible with a ketogenic diet (see our book *Paleo-Ketogenic: The Why and the How*).

Ketosis

Ketosis is a metabolic state where the majority of the body's energy supply is derived from ketone bodies in the blood. This is in contrast with a state of glycolysis where blood glucose provides the majority of the energy supply.

Ketoacidosis

Diabetic ketoacidosis is a potentially life-threatening complication caused by a lack of insulin in the body. This may occur if the body is unable to use blood sugar (glucose) as a source of fuel. Instead, the body breaks down fat as an alternative source of fuel and because of the severity of the situation in diabetic ketoacidosis, this can lead to a dangerously high build-up of ketones.

Ketosis, the breaking down of fat, is desirable and an entirely different thing.

Keto-adaptation

Keto-adaptation is being able to switch from burning sugar and carbs as a source of fuel to burning fat and fibre, giving the individual much longer-lasting energy and greater stamina.

Ketogenic hypoglycaemia – also known as 'keto flu'

This is described in detail in Chapter 5.

Leaky gut

Leaky gut means that substances which should be held in the gut leak out through the gut wall. This causes many problems:

- Hydrogen ions (i.e. acid) cannot be concentrated in the stomach, leading to hypochlorhydria – a lack of stomach acid. This causes malabsorption of minerals and vitamin B12. Hypochlorhydria is a major risk factor for fermenting gut since acid helps to sterilise the upper gut. It also is an essential part of protein digestion.
- Allergy - Normally one expects foods to be completely broken down into amino acids (from protein), essential fatty acids and glycerol (from fats) and single sugars, or 'monosaccharides' (from carbohydrates). The undigested foods stay in the gut and the small, digested molecules pass through the gut wall into the portal bloodstream and on to the liver where they are dealt with. However, leaky gut means food particles get absorbed before they have been properly digested. This means large food molecules get into the bloodstream. These large molecules are 'interesting' to the immune system, which may mistake them for viruses and/or bacteria. In this event, it may attack these harmless molecules, either with antibodies or directly with immune cells. This causes inflammation. Inflammation in the gut causes diseases of the gut. Inflammation elsewhere can cause almost any symptom you care to mention. It may switch on allergy and/or auto-immunity – that is, it is potentially a disease-amplifying process.
- Another problem with small, digested molecules or polypeptides getting into the bloodstream is that these molecules may be biologically active. Some of them act as hormone mimics, which can affect levels of glucose in the blood or blood pressure. This is akin to throwing a handful of sand into a finely tuned machine – it makes a real mess of homeostatic (balancing) mechanisms of controlling body activities.

Magnesium

Magnesium is an essential mineral required for at least 300 different enzyme systems in the body. It is centrally involved in the energy delivery systems of the body – that is, the mitochondria.

Red blood cell levels of magnesium are almost invariably low in my ME patients and very many benefit from magnesium by injection.

I believe that a low red-cell magnesium is a symptom of mitochondrial failure. It is the job of mitochondria to produce ATP for cell metabolism, and about 40% of all mitochondrial output goes into maintaining calcium/magnesium and sodium/potassium ion pumps. I suspect that when mitochondria fail, these pumps malfunction and therefore calcium leaks into cells and magnesium leaks out. This, of course, compounds the underlying mitochondrial failure because calcium is toxic to mitochondria and magnesium necessary for normal mitochondrial function. This is just one of the many vicious cycles we see in patients with fatigue syndromes. The reason for giving magnesium by injection is in order to reduce the work of the calcium/magnesium ion pump by reducing the concentration gradient across cell membranes.

Malabsorption

The job of the gut is to absorb the goodness from food. To do this, it first has to reduce food particles to a size which allows the digestive enzymes to get at them; then it has to provide the correct acidity then alkalinity for enzymes to work, produce the necessary enzymes and emulsifying agent (bile salts), and move the food along the gut. Lastly, the large bowel allows growth of bacteria for a final digestive/fermentative process and water extraction.

The gut has a particularly difficult job because it has to identify foods that are safe from potentially dangerous microbes (most are not dangerous but positively beneficial). This explains why 90% of the immune system is associated with the gut. The inoculation of the gut with these gut-friendly microbes takes place in the first few minutes following birth.

Anything which goes wrong with any of these processes can cause malabsorption. Malabsorption means that the body does not get the raw materials for normal everyday work and repair. Consequently, there is the potential for much more to go wrong.

Metabolic inflexibility

Metabolic inflexibility is the condition that arises when the body cannot switch from burning sugars and starches as its fuel source to running on fibres and fats. This is the opposite of keto-adaptation – that is, the metabolic condition which arises when the body is powering itself from fat and ketones. This inflexibility can give rise to ketogenic hypoglycaemia – see above and Chapter 5.

Metabolic syndrome

This is the clinical picture which arises when the body powers itself predominantly with sugars and carbohydrates. There is a loss of control over blood sugar levels. The conventional definition of metabolic syndrome only occurs in an advanced state of such – that is, when there is a combination of abdominal (central) obesity (i.e. being apple shaped), high blood pressure, high fasting sugar, high triglycerides and low levels of friendly high-density lipoprotein (HDL). My advice is not to wait for these nasty and damaging features to emerge, but to tackle the metabolic syndrome early by eating a PK diet as described in this book.

Minerals

You could argue that we all die ultimately from mineral and vitamin deficiencies. People who traditionally live to a great age are often found living in areas watered by streams from glaciers. Glaciers are lakes of ice which have spent the previous few thousand years crunching up rocks. Therefore, the waters coming from the glaciers are rich in minerals. This is used not just to drink but to irrigate crops and to bathe in. These people therefore have had excellent levels of micronutrients throughout life. Given the right raw materials, things do not go wrong in the body and ageing is slowed. For example:

- Low magnesium and selenium are a risk factor for heart disease
- Low selenium increases the risk of cancer
- Copper is necessary to make elastic tissue – deficiency causes weaknesses in arteries, leading to aneurysms
- Low chromium increases the risk of diabetes
- Good antioxidant status (vitamins A, C, E and selenium) slows the ageing process
- The superoxide dismutase enzymes (which counteract oxygen free radicals) require zinc, copper and manganese to function
- Iodine is necessary to make thyroid hormones and is highly protective against breast disease
- The immune system needs a huge range of minerals to work well, especially zinc, selenium and magnesium
- Boron is highly protective against arthritis
- Magnesium is required in at least 300 enzyme systems
- Zinc is needed for normal brain development – a deficiency at a critical stage of development causes dyslexia
- Any deficiency of selenium, zinc, copper or magnesium can cause infertility
- Iron prevents anaemia
- Molybdenum is necessary to detox sulphites.

The secret of success is to copy Nature. Civilisation and Western diets have brought great advantages, but at the same time are responsible for escalating death rates from cancer, heart disease and dementia. I want the best of both worlds. I like my warm kitchen, fridge, wood-burning cooker, computer and telly, but I want to eat and live in the environment in which primitive man thrived.

Nickel (Ni)

Nickel is a nasty, toxic metal and a known carcinogen. It is one of the metals we see most commonly in toxicity tests – it appears stuck onto DNA, stuck on to translocator protein and is often present in blood at high levels. Nickel is a problem because biochemically it 'looks' like zinc. Zinc deficiency is very common in people eating Western diets, and so if the body needs zinc and it is not there, it will use look-alike nickel instead. But nickel does not do the job and, indeed, gets in the way of normal biochemistry. Zinc is an essential co-factor in many enzyme systems, from alcohol dehydrogenase to zinc carboxypeptidase, and so there is enormous potential for harm from nickel.

Nickel sensitivity is very common and often diagnosed from rashes from jewellery, zips, watches etc. What we know from people with chemical sensitivity is that they often have toxic loads of those things they are sensitive to. So, nickel sensitivity often equates with nickel toxicity.

Nickel is unavoidable if you live a Western lifestyle. Many industrial and other processes release nickel into the atmosphere:

- Stainless steel contains 14% nickel; this includes cookware and eating utensils. Use cast iron pans, glass or ceramic.
- Jewellery – used because it is such a versatile, malleable metal. It is well-absorbed with piercing.
- Catalytic converters in cars release fine particulate nickel into the atmosphere – so fine that it cannot be filtered out by the lining of the bronchus, so it is well-absorbed by inhalation and easily gets into blood vessels. Here it triggers inflammation and arterial disease.
- Cigarette smoke.
- Medical prostheses such as artificial hip joints.

Organophosphate (OP) poisoning

OP poisoning is a remarkably common but under-diagnosed problem because we are all constantly exposed to organophosphates, including glyphosate – this (Round-up is the best-known product) is generally regarded as safe, but this is not so.

Different people have different symptoms of OP poisoning and these symptoms depend partly on how much OP they have been exposed to, whether they have had single massive exposure or chronic sub-lethal exposure, whether it has been combined with other chemicals, and how good their body is at coping with toxic chemicals. Symptoms divide into the following categories:

- **No obvious symptoms at all** – A government-sponsored study at the Institute of Occupational Medicine, UK, that looked at farmers who regularly handled OPs but who were complaining of no symptoms, showed that they suffered from mild brain damage. Their ability to think clearly and problem solve was impaired.
- **Sheep dip 'flu (mild acute poisoning)** – This is a 'flu-like illness which follows exposure

to OPs. Sometimes the farmer just has a bit of a headache, feels unusually tired or finds s/he can't think clearly. This may just last a few hours to a few days and the sufferer recovers completely. Most sufferers do not realise that they have been poisoned and put any symptoms down to a hard day's work. It can occur after dipping, but some farmers will get symptoms after the slightest exposure, such as visiting markets and inhaling OP fumes from fleeces.

- **Acute organophosphate poisoning** – This is the syndrome recognised by doctors and Poisons Units. Symptoms occur within 24 hours of exposure and include collapse, breathing problems, sweating, diarrhoea, vomiting, excessive salivation, heart dysrhythmias, extreme anxiety etc. Treatment is with atropine. You have to have a large dose of OP to have this effect (such as, drink some of the dip!) and so this syndrome is rarely seen.
- **Intermediate syndrome** – This occurs one to three weeks after exposure and is characterised by weakness of shoulder, neck and upper leg muscles. It is rarely diagnosed because it goes unrecognised.
- **Long-term chronic effects** – These symptoms develop in some susceptible individuals. They can either occur following a single massive exposure, or after several years of regular sub-lethal exposure to OPs. Essentially there is an acceleration of the normal ageing process, with arterial disease, heart disease, cancer and dementia presenting at a young age.

Osteoporosis

Osteoporosis is a modern disease of Western society. Primitive societies eating PK diets do not suffer from osteoporosis. So, the underlying principle for avoiding osteoporosis is that we should mimic primitive cultures eating a PK diet and living as toxin-free a life as possible. This does not mean you need to run around half naked in a rabbit-skin loin cloth depriving yourself of the pleasures of 21st century Western life. We need to cherry-pick from the good things of all civilisations.

To make good quality bone you need the raw materials (PK diet and supplements), the ability to absorb minerals (an acid stomach) and the drive to lay these down in bone (exercise, vitamin D). I have collected before and after bone density scans of 14 patients doing these regimes. In all cases, the bone density has remained the same or increased. So, whilst the numbers are small the statistics are powerful.

Dairy products and calcium supplements alone make osteoporosis worse. This is because calcium in isolation blocks the absorption of other essential minerals, such as magnesium. Vitamin D is the key to calcium – it promotes the absorption of calcium (and magnesium) and ensures its deposition in bone.

The medical profession would have us believe that the only important constituent of bone is calcium. Actually, bone is made up of many different minerals, including magnesium, calcium, potassium, boron, silicon, manganese, iron, zinc, copper, chromium, strontium and maybe others. For its formation it also requires a whole range of vitamins, essential fatty acids and amino acids.

Pain

Although pain seems like 'a pain', actually it is essential for our survival. Pain protects us from ourselves. It prevents us from damaging our bodies. Indeed, people who are born with no pain perception look as if they have been traumatised – they are covered in cuts, bruises and sores, because they are unaware that they are damaging themselves. Pain is the local method of avoiding damage – it makes us protect the affected part of the body and keep it still so that healing and repair can take place. If pain becomes more generalised, then it is accompanied by fatigue. What this means is that chronic pain and chronic fatigue go hand in hand and therefore so should treatment. We learn through experience what is painful; this makes us avoid those painful experiences and therefore protects our bodies.

Although it is desirable to learn about pain, this can also cause problems because if the underlying causes of the pain are not identified we 'learn' more pain. In the ideal situation, we damage our bodies with say a cut or bruise and the local pain makes us care for that damaged area by protecting it and keeping it still so that healing and repair can take place. With healing the pain goes. If the root source of the pain is not identified, it creates a problem because then the pain increases. The body naturally thinks that increasing pain means we will take more care, identify the source of the pain, keep the limb more still and therefore the body winds up the pain signal to try to elicit the appropriate response. Effectively we learn to feel more pain because there is an upgrading of this pain response. This is not a psychological effect – this actually occurs within the cells themselves. This makes it very important to identify causes of pain early on in any disease process and allow time for healing and repair, otherwise the pain will get worse.

Pancreatic function

The pancreas is a large gland which lies behind the stomach and upper gut. It has two major functions of clinical importance. Firstly, it acts as an endocrine organ to produce insulin and other hormones essential for the control of blood sugar. Secondly, it has an exocrine function to produce enzymes essential for the digestion of food. These enzymes include those to digest proteins, fats and starches, and to work best they need an alkali environment as is found in the small intestine courtesy of the pancreas. When food is present in the duodenum and jejunum (the first two sections of the small intestine), the gall bladder contracts, sending in a bolus of bile salts which combine with bicarbonate and pancreatic enzymes to allow digestion to take place.

If the pancreas does not produce sufficient digestive enzymes and bicarbonate, then foods will not be digested. This can lead to problems downstream. Firstly, foods may be fermented instead of being digested and this can produce the symptom of bloating due to wind, together with metabolites such as various alcohols, hydrogen sulphide and other toxic compounds. Secondly, foods are not fully broken down so they cannot be absorbed, and this can result in malabsorption.

Where there is severe pancreatic dysfunction, it is obvious because the stools themselves become greasy and fatty, foul smelling, bulky and difficult to flush away. Where there is malabsorption of fat, there will be malabsorption of essential fatty acids such as the omega-3 and omega-6 fatty acids, and there will be malabsorption of fat-soluble vitamins such as vitamins A, D, E and K.

If foods are poorly digested, this results in large antigenically interesting molecules appearing downstream, which alerts the immune system and could switch on allergies – that is, poor digestion of food is a risk factor for allergy.

Where there is poor pancreatic function digestive aids can be very helpful. I use pancreatic enzymes together with magnesium carbonate 90 minutes after food (not with food since we need a 90-minute window of time of acidity for stomach function). High-dose pancreatic enzymes have revolutionised the treatment of cystic fibrosis.

Probiotics

In a normal situation, free from antiseptics, antibiotics, high-carbohydrate diets, bottle feeding, hormones and other such accoutrements of modern western life, the gut microbiome is safe. Babies start life in their mother's womb with a sterile gut (although interestingly there is some evidence that their gut becomes inoculated before birth through transfer of microbes across the placenta). During the process of birth, they become inoculated with bacteria from the birth canal and perineum. These bacteria are largely bacteroides which cannot survive for more than a few minutes outside the human gut. This inoculation is enhanced through breast-feeding because the first milk, namely colostrum, is a highly desirable substrate for these bacteria to flourish. We now know that this is an essential part of immune programming. Indeed, 90% of the immune system is gut associated.

These essential probiotics programme the immune system so that they accept them and learn what is beneficial. A healthy gut microbiome therefore is highly protective against invasion of the gut by other strains of bacteria or viruses. The problem is there is no probiotic on the market that supplies bacteroides for the above reasons. If we eat probiotics which have been artificially cultured, for a short while the levels of these probiotics in the gut do increase. However, as soon as we stop eating them, levels taper off and may disappear. Ideally for bacteria to be accepted into the normal gut and remain, they have to be programmed first through somebody else's gut (in this case, mother's).

So, when it comes to repleting gut flora, there are two ways that we can go about this – either we can take probiotics very regularly (and the cheapest way to do this is to grow your own probiotics) or to take bacteroides directly. Indeed, this latter technique is well established in the treatment of *Clostridium difficile* (a normally fatal gastroenteritis in humans) and interestingly in idiopathic (of unknown origin) diarrhoea in horses. In the latter case, horses are inoculated with the bacteria from the gut of another horse. These ideas have been developed further by Dr Thomas Borody with his ideas on faecal bacteriotherapy, which can provide a permanent cure in cases of ulcerative colitis, severe constipation, *Clostridium difficile* infection and pseudomembranous colitis. The reason this technique works so well is because the most abundant bacteria in the large bowel, bacteroides, cannot survive outside the human gut and cannot be given by any other route.

The gut microbiome is extremely stable and difficult to change. Therefore, if you are going to take probiotics, you have to be prepared to take them for the long term. Many preparations on the market are ineffective. Those found to be most effective are those milk ferments and live yoghurts where the product is freshly made. It is not really surprising. Keeping bacteria alive is difficult and it is not surprising that they do not survive dehydration and storage at room temperature. So, your best chance of eating live viable bacteria is to buy live yoghurts or drinks. These can be easily grown at home, just as one would make home-made yoghurt. If you cannot grow easily from a culture, then it suggests that the culture is not active, so this is a good test of what is and is not viable (see Chapter 18).

Sleep

Humans evolved to sleep when it is dark and wake when it is light. Sleep is a form of hibernation when the body shuts down in order to repair damage done through use, to conserve energy and to hide from predators. The normal sleep pattern that evolved in hot climates is to sleep, keep warm and conserve energy during the cold nights and then to sleep again in the afternoons when it is too hot to work and to hide away from the midday sun. As humans migrated away from the Equator, the sleep pattern had to change with the seasons and as the lengths of the days changed.

After the First World War a strain of Spanish 'flu swept through Europe killing 50 million people worldwide. Some people sustained neurological damage and for some this virus wiped out their sleep centre in the brain. This meant they were unable to sleep at all. All these unfortunate people were dead within two weeks, and this was the first solid scientific evidence that sleep was as essential for life as food and water. Indeed, all living creatures require a regular 'sleep' (or period of quiescence) during which time healing and repair take place. You must put as much work into your sleep as your diet. Without a good night's sleep on a regular basis all other interventions are undermined.

Syndrome X

Syndrome X is a pre-diabetic state, also known as 'metabolic syndrome', when blood sugar levels see-saw between too high and too low in the presence of excessively high levels of insulin.

Thyroid hormones and 'reverse T3'

T4 (named because it contains four iodine atoms) is synthesised in the thyroid gland but is relatively inactive compared to T3 (three iodine atoms). T4 is activated to T3 in the peripheral tissues according to local needs. This process requires selenium and zinc. There is a further mechanism for controlling the local action of T3. In conditions of stress (such as starvation, infection, organ failures) more is converted to reverse T3, thereby blocking the effect of T3. This occurs locally so energy can be diverted to those organs essential for dealing with that stressed state. Poor conversion of inactive T4 to active T3 is one of the four types of hypothyroidism - T3 hypothyroidism. When testing thyroid function, always measure free T4 and free T3, NOT T4 and T3. The T4 and T3 levels are affected by protein binding and so are unreliable measures of the actual 'available' levels of hormones.

Thyroid stimulating hormone (TSH)

Thyroid-stimulating hormone (also known as thyrotropin, or thyrotropic hormone) is produced by the pituitary gland. It stimulates the thyroid gland to produce thyroid hormones.

Thyroid glandular (TG)

These are glandular extracts that come from the thyroid glands of animals, usually cows, but sometimes sheep and pigs. They contain dried and ground-up raw animal thyroid glandular tissues or extracts of those tissues. Other glandulars derive from the adrenals, pituitary, ovaries, testes and pancreas.

Thyrotoxicosis and hyperthyroidism (overactive thyroid)

Thyrotoxicosis is the name for when you have too much thyroid hormone in your body. Hyperthyroidism is a type of thyrotoxicosis and happens specifically when your thyroid gland both produces and releases excess thyroid hormone. Thyrotoxicosis happens when you have too much thyroid hormone in your body in general. You could have too much thyroid hormone from taking too much thyroid medication, for example. This would be thyrotoxicosis, not hyperthyroidism. Some causes of hyperthyroidism include:

- Graves' disease (see page 188)
- Toxic nodular goitre (also called 'multinodular goitre') – Hyperthyroidism here is caused by toxic nodular goitre, a condition in which one or more nodules of the thyroid become(s) overactive.
- (Sub-acute) thyroiditis (SAT) – Thyroiditis causes **temporary hyperthyroidism**, usually followed by hypothyroidism, an underactive thyroid, as in Hashimoto's thyroiditis – see Chapters 1, 2, 6, 9 and 11 for more detail.

Toxins

Toxins are substances that are dangerous to the body because they inhibit normal metabolism, damage the structure of the body or are wasteful of its resources. Organophosphates, for example, inhibit the essential process of oxidative phosphorylation. Toxic metals can stick onto DNA and trigger cancer; they also stick on to proteins to trigger prion disorders. Products of the fermenting gut require energy and micronutrients for the liver to deal with them. Volatile organic compounds (VOCs) may need methylating to detoxify them, and this is a drain on folic acid and vitamin B12.

Toxins come from the outside world (exogenous) and the inside world (endogenous). Exogenous toxins include POPs (persistent organic pollutants), metals, radiation (most of this comes from the medical profession), toxic halides (fluorides, bromides) and many more. A major source of toxic stress is from prescription medication. Endogenous toxins come from the fermenting gut, natural toxins in foods (e.g. lectins, mycotoxins), breakdown products of normal metabolism, inflammation and other such. Modern Western lifestyles mean we are inevitably exposed to chemicals.

Yeast problems – including candida

Yeast is one of the common fermenting microbes in the upper gut and is part of the upper fermenting gut issue (see page 26). Yeast problems are an inevitable problem of Western diets, which are high in carbohydrates. The problem is worsened by antibiotics, the Pill and HRT.

Problems may arise initially because yeast numbers build up, sometimes to produce overt infections such as oral thrush, perineal thrush or skin tinea infections (ringworm, athlete's foot, fungal toenails, tinea etc). With chronic exposures there is the potential to sensitise to yeast and that causes much worse problems, characterised by itching, pain and inflammation. Psoriasis may be allergy to yeast; ditto chronic cystitis and interstitial cystitis.

References

Preface

1. Burton R. *The Anatomy of Melancholy.* First published 1621.
   www.gutenberg.org/files/10800/10800-h/10800-h.htm
2. Humphry GM. Report of a Committee of the Clinical Society Of London. *J Anat Physiol* 1886;
   20(Pt3): 546-547. www.ncbi.nlm.nih.gov/pmc/articles/PMC1288618/
3. Asher R. Myxoedematous madness. *Br Med J* 1949; 2(4627): 555–562.
   doi: doi.org/10.1136/bmj.2.4627.555 www.bmj.com/content/2/4627/555

Introduction: Do it yourself because your doctor won't

1. www.drmyhill.co.uk/wiki/Press_Release_re_my_Non_Compliance_Hearing_-_MPTS_-_
   Myhill_vs_GMC_Sept_28_to_Oct_1_2020

Chapter 1: Are you hypothyroid?

1. Arafah BM. Increased Need for Thyroxine in Women with Hypothyroidism during Estrogen
   Therapy. *N Engl J Med* 2001; 344:1743-1749.
   www.nejm.org/doi /10.1056/NEJM200106073442302
2. Panicker V. Genetics of Thyroid Function and Disease. *Clin Biochem Rev* 2011; 32(4):
   165–175. https://www.ncbi.nlm.nih.gov/ pmc/articles/PMC3219766/
3. Surks M. Lithium and the Thyroid. www.uptodate.com/contents/
   lithium-and-the-thyroid?search=lithium%20and%20the%20thyroid&source=search_result&se-
   lectedTitle=1~150&usage_type=default&display_rank=1 (Accessed 1 July 2022)

4. Keh-Chuan L. Amiodarone-induced thyroid disorders: a clinical review. *BMJ: Postgraduate Medical Journal* 2000; 76(893): 133-140. doi.org/10.1136/pmj.76.893.133

5. Bax ND, Lennard MS, Tucker GT. Effect of beta blockers on thyroid hormone. *Br Med J* 1980; 281(6250): 1283. doi: 10.1136/bmj.281.6250.1283

6. Vera-Lastra O, Navarro Ao, Dominguez MPC. Two Cases of Graves' Disease Following SARS-CoV-2 Vaccination: An Autoimmune/Inflammatory Syndrome Induced by Adjuvants. *Thyroid* 2021; 31(9): 1436-1439.
doi: 10.1089/thy.2021.0142 https://pubmed.ncbi.nlm.nih.gov/33858208/

7. Nishihara E, Ohye H, Amino N, et al. Clinical Characteristics of 852 Patients with Subacute Thyroiditis before Treatment. *Internal Medicine* 2008; 47(8): 725-729. doi.org/10.2169/internalmedicine.47.0740 www.jstage.jst.go.jp/article/internalmedicine/47/8/47_8_725/_article

8. Shoenfeld Y, Aron-Maor A. Vaccination and autoimmunity. Vaccinosis: A dangerous liaison? *J Autoimun* 2000; 14(1): 1-10. doi: 10.1006/jaut.1999.0346

9. Nossal GJV. Vaccination and autoimmunity. *JAI* 2000; 14: 15-22.

10. Shoenfeld Y, Aron-Maor A, Sherer Y. Vaccination as an additional player in the mosaic of autoimmunity. *Clin Exp Rheumatol* 2000; 18(2): `181-184. PMID: 10812488

11. Cohen AD, Shoenfeld Y. Vaccine-induced autoimmunity. *J Autoimmun* 1996; 9(6): 699-703. doi: 10.1006/jaut.1996.0091

11A. Rogerson SJ, Nye FJ. Hepatitis B vaccine associated with erythema nodosum and polyarthritis. *Br Med J* 1990; 301: 345. doi: https://doi.org/10.1136/bmj.301.6747.345

12. Haschulla E, Houvenagel E, Mingui A, Vincent G, Laine A. Reactive arthritis after hepatitis B vaccination. *J Rheumatol* 1990; 17: 1250-1251.

13. Biasi D, De Sandre G, Bambara LM, Carletto A, Caramaschi P, Zanoni G, Tridente G. A new case of reactive arthritis after hepatitis B vaccination. *Clin Exp Rheumatol* 1993; 11(2): 215. PMID: 8508565

14. Biasi D, Carletto A, Caramaschi P, Frigo A, Pacor ML, Bezzi D, Bambara LM. Rheumatological manifestations following hepatitis B vaccination. A report of 2 clinical cases (article in Italian). *Recenti Prog Med* 1994; 85(9): 438-440. PMID: 7938876

15. Gross K. Combe C, Kruger K, Schattenkirschner M. Arthritis after hepatitis B vaccination. Report of three cases. *Scand J Rheumatol* 1995; 24: 50-52. doi: 10.3109/03009749509095156.

16. Cathebras P, Cartry O, Lafage-Proust MH, et al. Arthritis, hypercalcemia and lytic bone lesions after hepatitis B vaccination. *J Rheumatol* 1996; 23: 558-560.

17. Maillefert JF, Sibilia J, Toussirot E, et al. Rheumatic disorders developed after hepatitis B vaccination. *Rheumatology* 1999; 38: 978-983. doi: 10.1093/rheumatology/38.10.978.

18. Grasland A, Le Maitre F, Pouchot J, et al. Adult-onset Still's disease after hepatitis A and B vaccination (article in French). *Rev Med Interne* 1998; 19(2): 134-136.
doi: 10.1016/s0248-8663(97)83425-x

19. Pope JE, Stevens A, Howson W, Bell DA. The development of rheumatoid arthritis after recombinant hepatitis B vaccination. *J Reumatol* 1998; 25(9): 1687-1693. PMID: 9733447

20. Tudela P, Marti S, Bonanl J. Systemic lupus erythematosus and vaccination against hepatitis B. *Nephron* 1992; 62(2): 236. doi: 10.1159/000187043

21. Finielz P, Lam-Kam-Sang LF. Systemic lupus erythematosus and thrombocytopenic purpura in two members of the same family. *Nephrol Dial Transplant* 1998; 13: 2420-2421.

22. Guiseriz J. Systemic lupus erythematosus following hepatitis B vaccine. *Nephron* 1996; 74: 441.

23. Mamoux V, Dumont C. Lupus erythemateux dissemine et vaccination contre l'hepatite B. *Arch Pediatr* 1994; 1: 307-308.

24. Grezard P, Chafi M, Philippot V, Perrot H, Faisant M. Cutaneoius lupus erythematosus and buccal aphthosis after hepatitis B vaccination in a 6-year-old child. *Ann Dermatol Venereol* 1996; 123: 657-659.

25. Weibel RE, Bemor DE. Chronic arthropathy and musculoskeletal symptoms associated with rubella vaccines. A review of 124 claims submitted to the National Vaccine Injury Compensation Program. *Arthritis Rheum* 1996; 39: 1529-1534.

26. Ray P, Black S, Shinefield H, et al. Risk of chronic arthropathy among women after rubella vaccination. Vaccine Safety Datalink Team. *JAMA* 1997; 278: 551-556.

27. Howson CP, Fineberg HV. Adverse events following pertussis and rubella vaccines. Summary of a report of the Institute of Medicine. *JAMA* 1992; 267; 392-396.

28. Howson CP, Katz M, Johnston RB Jr, Fineberg HV. Chronic arthritis after rubella vaccination. *Clin Infect Dis* 1992; 15: 307-312.

29. Mitchell LA, Tingle AJ, MacWilliam L, Horne C, Keown P, Gaur LK, Nepom GT. HLA-DR class II associations with rubella vaccine-induced joint manifestations. *J Infect Dis* 1998; 177: 5-12.

30. Mitchell LA, Tingle AJ, Grace M, Middleton P, Chalmers AC. Rubella virus vaccine associated arthropathy in postpartum immunized women: influence of preimmunization serologic status on development of joint manifestations. *J Rheumatol* 2000; 27: 418-423.

31. Nussinovitch M, Harel L, Varsano I. Arthritis after mumps and measles vaccination. *Arch Dis Child* 1995; 72: 348-349.

32. Thurairajan G, Hope-Ross MW, Situnayake RD, Murray PI. Polyarthropathy, orbital myositis and posterior scleritis: an unusual adverse reaction to influenza vaccine. *Br J Rheumatol* 1997; 36: 120-123.

33. Maillefert JF, Tonolli-Serabian I, Cherasse A, et al. Arthritis following combined vaccine against diphtheria, polyomyelitis and tetanus toxoid. *Clin Exp Rheumatol* 2000; 18: 255-256.

34. Adachi JA, D`Alessio FR, Ericsson CD. Reactive arthritis associated with typhoid vaccination in travellers: report of two cases with negative HLA-B27. *J Travel Med* 2000; 7: 35-36.

35. Older SA, Battafarano DF, Enzenauer RJ, Krieg AM. Can immunization precipitate connective tissue disease? Report of five cases of systemic lupus erythematosus and review of the literature. *Sem Arthritis Rheum* 1999; 29: 131-139.

36. Kennedy JR. Reactive arthritis: the result of an anti-idiotypic immune response to a bacterial lipopolysaccharide antigen where the idiotype has the immunological appearance of a synovial antigen. *Med Hypotheses* 2000; 54: 723-725.

37. Hogenesch H, Azcona-Olivera J, Scott-Montcrieff C, Snyder PW, Glickman LT. Vaccine-induced autoimmunity in the dog. *Adv Med Vet* 1999; 41: 733-747.

38. Akinosoglou K, Tzivaki I, Marangos M. Covid-19 vaccine and autoimmunity: Awakening the sleeping dragon. *Clin Immunol* 2021; 226: 108721. doi: 10.1016/j.clim.2021.108721

Chapter 2: Blood tests for the underactive thyroid

1. Mikulic M. Global pharmaceutical industry – statistics and facts. *Statista* 10 September 2021. www.statista.com/topics/1764/global-pharmaceutical-industry/

2. Blanchard K, Abrams BM. *What Your Doctor May Not Tell You About Hypothyroidism*. US: Grand Central Publishing; 2004.

3. Subclinical Hypothyroidism. In: *Encyclopedia of Endocrine Diseases* 2nd edition. Elsevier 2017. www.sciencedirect.com/topics/medicine-and-dentistry/subclinical-hypothyroidism

4. McEvoy S. Levothyroxine half-lfe – How long does it stay your system? *Drug Genius* 10 December 2020. https://druggenius.com/half-life/levothyroxine/ (Accessed 1 July 2022)

5. Melmed S, et al. Liothyrine. In: *Willians Textbook of Endocrinology* (13th Edition). Elsevier (Science Direct); 2016. www.sciencedirect.com/topics/pharmacology-toxicology-and-pharmaceutical-science/liothyronine (Accessed 22 July 2022)

6. Oxford University Hospitals. Thyroid Antibodies. www.ouh.nhs.uk/immunology/diagnostic-tests/tests-catalogue/thyroid-antibodies.aspx

7. Wahab F, Kearney E, Joseph S. The presence of thyroid peroxidase antibodies in Graves' disease is predictive of disease duration and relapse rates. *Endocrine Abstracts* 2013; 31: 367. www.endocrine-abstracts.org/ea/0031/ea0031p367

8. Mehananthan PB, et al. Antithyroid Peroxidase Antibodies in Multinodular Hashimoto's Thyroiditis Indicate a Variant Etiology. *J Thyroid Res* 2019; 2019: 4892329. www.ncbi.nlm.nih.gov/pmc/ articles/PMC6679885/

9. Dohee K. The Role of Vitamin D in Thyroid Diseases. *Int J Mol Sci* 2017; 18(9): 1949. www.ncbi.nlm.nih.gov/ pmc/articles/PMC5618598/

10. Lewis PJ. Iodine deficiency, not excess, is the cause of autoimmune thyroid disease. *BMJ Rapid Response* 2016; 352: i941. doi.org/10.1136/bmj.i941 www.bmj.com/content/352/bmj.i941/rr-2

11. Krysiak R, Szkrobka W, Okopien B. The Effect of Gluten-Free Diet on Thyroid Autoimmunity in Drug-Naïve Women with Hashimoto's Thyroiditis: A Pilot Study'. *Exp Clin Endocrinol Diabetes* 2019; 127(7): 417-422.
    doi: 10.1055/a-0653-7108 https://pubmed.ncbi.nlm.nih.gov/30060266/
12. Wentz I. Will Going Dairy Free to Reverse Your Hashimoto's. thyroidpharmacist.com 29 October 2021. https://thyroidpharmacist.com/articles/going-dairy-free-to-reverse-hashimotos/ (Accessed 1 July 2022).
13. Cojocaru M, Cojocaru IM, Silosi I. Multiple autoimmune syndrome. *Journal ListMaedica* 2010; 5(2); 132-134. PMID: 21977137
14. Stehouwer CDA, Weijenberg MP, van den Berg M, et al. Serum Homocysteine and Risk of Coronary Heart Disease and Cerebrovascular Disease in Elderly Men - A 10-Year Follow-Up. *Arteriosclerosis, Thrombosis and Vascular Biology* 1998; 18(12): 1895-1901.
    doi.org/10.1161/01.ATV.18.12.1895
15. Wu LL, Lu JT. Hyperhomocysteinemia is a risk factor for cancer and a new potential tumor marker. *Clin Chim Acta* 2002; 322(1-2): 218. https://pubmed.ncbi.nlm.nih.gov/12104077/
16. Leblhuber F, Walli J, Artner-Dworzak E, Vrecko K, et al. Hyperhomocysteinemia in dementia. *J Neural Transm* 2000; 107(12): 1469-1474.
    doi: 10.1007/s007020070010 https://pubmed.ncbi.nlm.nih.gov/11458999/
17. Strain JJ, Dowey L, Pentieva K, McNulty H. B-vitamins, homocysteine metabolism and CVD. *Proc Nutr Soc* 2004; 63(4): 597-603.
    doi: 10.1079/pns2004390 https://pubmed.ncbi.nlm.nih.gov/15831132/
18. Landon A. This is the heartwarming reason 'mind the gap' sounds so different at Embankment Station. Secret London 12 December 2019. https://secretldn.com/mind-the-gap-embank-ment-station/ (Accessed 1 July 2022)
19. Original Mind the Gap Announcement – Northern Line Embankment. 20 April 2017. www.youtube.com/watch?v=QExoX4ls9OM

Chapter 3: Before you start a trial of thyroid glandular (TG)

1. Technically, the Sun Still Never Sets Over the British Empire. Foreign Policy 23 July 2013. https://foreignpolicy.com/2013/07/23/technically-the-sun-still-never-sets-over-the-british-empire/ (Accessed 1 July 2022)
2. Kalla P. Introductory Psychology Blog (S14)_C. Why you shouldn't wear new clothes on a Tuesday. Penn State University 5 February 2014.
   https://sites.psu.edu/intropsychsp14n3/2014/02/05/why-you-shouldnt-wear-new-clothes-on-a-tuesday/ (Accessed 1 July 2022)

3. University of Reading. Glenn Gibson. www.reading.ac.uk/food/about/staff/g-r-gibson.aspx
4. Dykens JA, et al. Drug-induced mitochondrial dysfunction: An Emerging Model for Idiosyncratic Drug Toxicity. *Expert Rev Mol Diagnostics* 2007; 7: 161. www.mitoaction.org/wp-content/uploads/2019/04/Slides-Drug-Toxicity-and-Mitochondria-Dykens.pdf
5. Millan IS, et al Chronic lactate exposure decreases mitochondrial function by inhibition of fatty acid uptake and cardiolipin alterantions in neonatal rat cardiomyocytes. *Front Nutr* 2022; 9: 809485.

Chapter 4: The adrenal gearbox

1. Collaborative Group on Hormonal Factors in Breast Cancer. Type and timing of menopausal hormone therapy and breast cancer risk: individual participant meta-analysis of the worldwide epidemiological evidence. *Lancet* 2019; 394(10204): 1159-1168. https://www.thelancet.com/journals/lancet/article/PIIS0140-6736(19)31709-X/fulltext

Chapter 5: How to trial thyroid glandular (TG)

1. Lindholm J, Laurberg P. Hypothyroidism and Thyroid Substitution: Historical Aspects. *Journal of Thyroid Research* 2011; 2011: 809341. www.hindawi.com/journals/jtr/2011/809341/
2. Murray GR. The life-history of the first case of myxoedema treated by thyroid extract. *Br Med J* 1920; 1(3089): 359–360. doi: 10.1136/bmj.1.3089.359 www.ncbi.nlm.nih.gov/pmc/articles/PMC2337775/
3. Vermiglio F, Lo Presti VP, Moleti M, et al. Attention Deficit and Hyperactivity Disorders in the Offspring of Mothers Exposed to Mild-Moderate Iodine Deficiency: A Possible Novel Iodine Deficiency Disorder in Developed Countries. *Journal of Clinical Endocrinology & Metabolism* 2004; 89(12): 6054–6060. https://academic.oup.com/jcem/article/89/12/6054/2844344

Chapter 6: How and why we become hypothyroid

1. Eastman CJ, Zimmermann MB. The Iodine Deficiency Disorders. [Updated 2018 Feb 6]. In: Feingold KR, Anawalt B, Boyce A, et al, Eds. *Endotext*. South Dartmouth (MA): MDText.com, Inc.; 2000. www.ncbi.nlm.nih.gov/books/NBK285556/
2. Ehrenfeld M, Tincani A, Andreoli L, et al. Covid-19 and autoimmunity. *Autoimmun Rev* 2020; 19(8): 102597. doi: 10.1016/j.autrev.2020.102597
3. Janegova A, Janega P, Rychly B, et al. The role of Epstein-Barr virus infection in the development of autoimmune thyroid diseases. *Endokrynologia Polska* 2015; 66(2): #39714. https://

References

journals.viamedica.pl/endokrynologia_polska/article/view/EP.2015.0020/29453

4. Ruggeri RM, et al. SARS-COV-2-related immune-inflammatory thyroid disorders: facts and perspectives. *Expert Rev Clin Immunol* 2021: 1–23. www.ncbi.nlm.nih.gov/pmc/articles/PMC8182818/

5. Catapani WR, et al. A patient with hepatitis B, antimicrosomal antibodies, and autoimmune hypothyroidism. *Postgraduate Medical Journal* 1996; : 752-753. https://pmj.bmj.com/content/postgradmedj/72/854/752.full.pdf

6. Pastore F, et al. Hepatitis C virus infection and thyroid autoimmune disorders: A model of interactions between the host and the environment. *World J Hepatol* 2016; 8(2): 83–91. www.ncbi.nlm.nih.gov/pmc/articles/PMC4716530/

7. Rehman MU, et al. The Association of Subacute Thyroiditis with COVID-19: a Systematic Review. *SN Compr Clin Med* 2021: 1–13. www.ncbi.nlm.nih.gov/pmc/articles/PMC8082479/

8. Desailloud R, Hober D. Viruses and thyroiditis: an update. *Virol J* 2009; 6: 5. www.ncbi.nlm.nih.gov/pmc/articles/PMC2654877/

9. Pekcici R, Kavlakoglu B, Yilmaz, et al. Effects of lead on thyroid functions in lead-exposed workers. *Central European Journal of Medicine* 2010; 5: 215-218. https://link.springer.com/article/10.2478/s11536-009-0092-8

10. Urinyova M, Uhnakova I, Serbin R, et al. The relation between human exposure to mercury and thyroid hormone status. *Biol Trace Elem Res* 2012; 148(3): 281-291. doi: 10.1007/s12011-012-9382-0 https://pubmed.ncbi.nlm.nih.gov/22426797/

11. Chen A, Kim SS, Chung E, Dietrich KN. Thyroid hormones in relation to lead, mercury and cadmium exposure in the National Health and Nutrition Examination Survey, 2007-2008. *Envrion Health Perspect* 2013; 121(2): 181-186. doi: 10.1289/ehp.1205239 www.ncbi.nlm.nih.gov/pmc/articles/PMC3569681/

12. Sarne D. Effects of the Environment, Chemicals and Drugs on Thyroid Function. *Endotext* 27 September 2016. www.ncbi.nlm.nih.gov/books/NBK285560/

13. Maskall K. Flame retardants and toxic furnishings. Killing us softly. *Pledging Change* 20 December 20118. https://pledgingforchange.com/social-responsibility/flame-retardants-and-toxic-furnishings-killing-us-softly.php

14. Kramer AB, et al. Familial occurrence of subacute thyroiditis associated with human leukocyte antigen-B35. *Thyroid* 2004; 14(7): 544-547. https://pubmed.ncbi.nlm.nih.gov/15307945/

15. Blick C, Nguyen M, Jialal I. Thyrotoxicosis. *StatPearls* 28 September 2021. www.ncbi.nlm.nih.gov/books/NBK482216/ (Accepted 1 July 2022)

16. Knezevic J, et al. Thyroid-Gut-Axis: How Does the Microbiota Influence Thyroid Function? *Nutrients* 2020; 12(6): 1769. www.ncbi.nlm.nih.gov/pmc/articles/PMC7353203/

17. Mindd Foundation. Environmental Toxins and their Role in Thyroid Diseases.

https://mindd.org/environmental-toxins-thyroid-diseases/ (Accessed 29 June 2022)

18. Acconcia F, Pallottini V, Marino M. Molecular mechanisms of action of BPA. *Dose Response 2015; 13(4): Acconcia F, Pallottini V, Marino M. Molecular mechanisms of action of BPA. Dose Response* 2015; 13(4). doi: 10.1177/1559325815610582.

19. Bajaj JK, Salwan P, Salwan S. Various possible toxicants involved in thyroid dysfunction: A review. *J Clin Diagn Res* 2016; 10(1): FE01-3. doi: 10.7860/JCDR/2016/15195.7092.

20. Brent GA. Environmental exposures and autoimmune thyroid disease. *Thyroid* 2010; 20(7): 755-761. doi: 10.1089/thy.2010.1636.

21. Ferrari SM, Fallahi P, Antonelli A, Benvenga S. Environmental issues in thyroid diseases. *Front. Endocrinol* 2017. 10(3389).

22. Konieczna A, Rutkowska A, Rachoń D. Health risk exposure to Bisphenol A (BPA). *Rocz Panstw Zakl Hig* 2015; 66(1): 5-11.

23. Vojdani A. A potential link between environmental triggers and autoimmunity. *Autoimmune Dis* 2014; 2014(437231).

24. Dutta P, Kamath SS, Bhalla A, et al. Effects of acute organophosphate poisoning on pituitary target gland hormones at admission, discharge and three months after poisoning: A hospital based pilot study. *Indian Journal of Endocrinology and Metabolism* 2015; 19(1): 116-123. doi: 10.4103/2230-8210.131771

25. Booij HA, et al. Pituitary dysfunction and association with fatigue in stroke and other acute brain injury. *Endocr Connect* 2018; 7(6): R223–R237. www.ncbi.nlm.nih.gov/pmc/articles/PMC6000755/

26. National Organization for Rare Diseases (NORD). Sheehan Syndrome. Rare Disease Database 2018 https://rarediseases.org/rare-diseases/sheehan-syndrome/ (Accessed 29 June 2022)

27. Singh BJ, Yen PM. A clinician's guide to understanding resistance to thyroid hormone due to receptor mutations in the TRα and TRβ isoforms. *Clinical Diabetes and Endocrinology* 2017; 3: 8: https://clindiabetesendo.biomedcentral.com/articles/10.1186/s40842-017-0046-z

28. National Organization for Rare Diseases (NORD). Sheehan Syndrome. Rare Disease Database 2018 https://rarediseases.org/rare-diseases/sheehan-syndrome/ (Accessed 29 June 2022)

Chapter 7: What happens if the diagnosis of hypothyroidism is missed?

1. Acheson D. *1089 and All That.* www.amazon.co.uk/1089-All-That-Journey-Mathematics/dp/0199590028

Chapter 8: Thyroid myths

1. Rong H, et al. Elevated Homocysteine Levels Associated with Atrial Fibrillation and Recurrent Atrial Fibrillation. *Int Heart J* 2020; 61(4): 705-712. https://pubmed.ncbi.nlm.nih.gov/32727999/

2. DiNicolantonio JJ, O'Keefe JH, Wilson W. Subclinical magnesium deficiency: a principal driver of cardiovascular disease and a public health crisis. *Open Heart* 2018; 5(1): e000668. doi:10.1136/openhrt-2017-000668

3. Michaëlsson K, Wolk A, Lanenskiold S, et al.Milk intake and risk of mortality and fractures in women and men: cohort studies. *BMJ* 2014; 349: g6015.
 doi: https://doi.org/10.1136/bmj.g6015

4. Singh J, Rani S, Parida A. Generation of piezoelectricity from the human body. 2014 *Annual International Conference on Emerging Research Areas: Magnetics, Machines and Drives* (AICERA/iCMMD) 2014; 400: 660. https://ieeexplore.ieee.org/document/6908277

5. Dean W. Strontium: Breakthrough Against Osteoporosis. WorldHealth.net 5 May 2004. www.worldhealth.net/news/strontium_breakthrough_against_osteoporo/

6. Prescribing Advice GPs. Strontium ranelate discontinued. 13 June 2017. www.prescriber.org.uk/2017/06/strontium-ranelate-discontinued/

Chapter 9: How we starve, destroy and poison the thyroid

1. O'Kane SM, et al. Micronutrients, iodine status and concentrations of thyroid hormones: a systematic review. *Nutr Rev* 2018; 76(6): 418-431. https://pubmed.ncbi.nlm.nih.gov/29596650/

2. The American Thyroid Association. 'Q and A' page. May 2007 www.thyroid.org/patient-thyroid-information/what-are-thyroid-problems/q-and-a-autoim-mune-thyroiditis/

3. Angum F, Khan T, Kaler J, et al. The Prevalence of Autoimmune Disorders in Women: A Narrative Review. *Cureus* 2020; 12(5): e8094. doi: 10.7759/cureus.8094

4. Cojocaru M, Cojocaru IM, Silosi I. Multiple autoimmune syndrome. *Journal ListMaedica* 2010; 5(2); 132-134. PMID: 21977137

5. Schwalfenberg GK. Solar Radiation and Vitamin D: Mitigating Environmental Factors in Autoimmune Disease. *Journal of Environmental and Public Health* 2012; 2012: 619381. www.hindawi.com/journals/jeph/2012/619381/

6. Soriano A, Butnaru D, Shoenfeld Y. Long-term inflammatory conditions following silicone exposure: the expanding spectrum of the autoimmune/ inflammatory syndrome induced by adjuvants (ASIA). *Clin Exp Rheumatol* 2014; 32(2): 151-154. https://pubmed.ncbi.nlm. nih.gov/24739519/

7. Colaris MJL, de Boer M, van der Hulst RR, Tervaert JWC. Two hundred cases of ASIA syndrome following silicone implants: a comparative study of 30 years and a review of current literature. *Immunol Res* 2017; 65(1): 120–128. https://pubmed.ncbi.nlm .nih.gov/27406737/

8. Draborg HA, Duus K, Houen G. Epstein-Barr virus in systemic autoimmune diseases. *Clinical Dev Immunology* 2013; 2013: 535738. www.ncbi.nlm.nih.gov/pmc/articles/PMC3766599/

9. Bagert BA. Epstein-Barr virus in multiple sclerosis. *Current Neurology and Neuroscience Reports* 2009; 9(5): 405-410. www.ncbi.nlm.nih.gov/pubmed/19664371

10. Hjalgrim H, Friborf J, Melbye M. The epidemiology of EBV and its association with malignant disease. In: Arvin A, Campadelli-Fium G, Mocarski E, et al (Eds). *Human Herpes Viruses: Biology, Therapy, and Immunoprophylaxis*. Cambridge: Cambridge University Press; 2007. www.ncbi.nlm.nih.gov/books/NBK47424/

11. Rashid T, Wilson C, Ebringer A. The Link between Ankylosing Spondylitis, Crohn's Disease, *Klebsiella, and Starch Consumption. Clin Dev Immunol* 2013; 2013: 872632. doi: 10.1155/2013/872632

12. Winzelberg GG, Gore J, Yu D, et al. Aspergillus flavus as a cause of thyroiditis in an immuno-suppressed host. *Johns Hopkins Med J* 1979; 144(3): 90-93. https://pubmed.ncbi.nlm.nih.gov/430949/

13. Rotter BA, Thompson BK, Lessard M, et al. Influence of low-level exposure to Fusarium mycotoxins on selected immunological and hematological parameters in young swine. *Fundam Appl Toxicol* 1994; 23(1): 117-124. doi: 10.1006/faat.1994.1087. https://pubmed.ncbi.nlm.nih.gov/7958555/

14. Wentz I. Mold: A Potential Trigger of Hashimoto's. *Thyroid Pharmacist* 24 July 2019. https://thyroidpharmacist.com/articles/mold-potential-trigger-hashimotos/ (Accessed 1 July 2022)

15. Palmery M. Oral contraceptives and changes in nutritional requirements. *Eur Rev Med Pharmacol Sci*2013; 17(13): 1804-1813. https://pubmed.ncbi.nlm.nih.gov/23852908/

16. Institute of Medicine (US) Committee on Thyroid Screening Related to I-131 Exposure. Exposure of the American People to Iodine-131 from Nevada Nuclear-Bomb Tests: Review of the National Cancer Institute Report and Public Health Implications. Washington DC (US): National Academies Press; 1999. www.ncbi.nlm.nih.gov/books/NBK100844/

17. Pfeiffer CC, Hoffer Abram. Nutrition and Mental Illness: An orthomolecular approach to balancing body chemistry. Inner Traditions Bear and Company; 1988.

18. Messina M, Redmond G. Effects of soy protein and soybean isoflavones on thyroid function in healthy adults and hypothyroid patients: a review of the relevant literature. *Thyroid* 2006; 16(3): 249-258. doi: 10.1089/thy.2006.16.249

19. Genova Diagnostics. Comprehensive Urine Element Profile. www.gdx.net/uk/product/comprehensive-urine-element-toxin-testing-urine

Chapter 10: The hypothyroid child

1. Grant ECG, et al. Zinc deficiency in children with dyslexia. 1988; 296(6622): 607–609. www.ncbi.nlm.nih.gov/pmc/articles/PMC2545239/
2. Leung AM. Thyroid function in pregnancy. *J Trace Elem Med Biol* 2012; 26(0): 137–140. www.ncbi.nlm.nih.gov/pmc/articles/PMC3990259/
3. Turkel H. Medical Amelioration of Down's Syndrome Incorporating the Orthomolecular Approach. *Orthomolecular Psychiatry* 1975; 4(2): 102-115. http://orthomolecular.org/library/jom/1975/pdf/1975-v04n02-p102.pdf

Chapter 11: The hypothyroid female

1. Nygaard B. Hypothyroidism (primary). *BMJ Clin Evid* 2010; 2010: 0605. www.ncbi.nlm.nih.gov/pmc/articles/PMC2907600/
2. Rifkin L. Is the meaning of life to make babies' in *Scientific American. Scientific American* 24 March 2013. https://blogs.scientificamerican.com/guest-blog/is-the-meaning-of-your-life-to-make-babies/ (Accepted 1 July 2022)
3. United Nations Population Fund. Maternal Health. www.unfpa.org/maternal-health#read-more-expand (Accessed 1 July 2022)
4. Moulton VR. Sex Hormones in Acquired Immunity and Autoimmune Disease. *Front. Immunol* 04 October 2018. doi.org/10.3389/fimmu.2018.02279
5. Contraceptives Study Group (Williams WV, et al.) Petition on Hormonal Contraceptives. www.drmyhill.co.uk/drmyhill/images/a/a2/Citizens_Petition_Final_updated_version_June_2019.pdf
6. Collaborative Group on Hormonal Factors in Breast Cancer. Type and timing of menopausal hormone therapy [MHT] and breast cancer risk: individual participant meta-analysis of the worldwide epidemiological evidence. *The Lancet* 2019; 394(10204): 1159-1168. www.thelancet.com/journals/lancet/article/PIIS0140-6736(19)31709-X/fulltext
7. Chalabi M. Why is puberty starting younger? *The Guardian* 4 November 2013. www.theguardian.com/politics/2013/nov/04/why-is-puberty-starting-younger-precocious (Accessed 1 February 2022)
8. Wynn M, Wynn A. The menstrual cycle as indicator or prepregnancy care. *Journal of Nutritional Medicine* 1991; 2(4): 387-398. doi.org/10.3109/13590849109084142
9. NICE Guideline. Fertility problems: assessment and treatment. NICE Clinical Guideline [CG156] 20 February 2013. www.nice.org.uk/guidance/cg156/chapter/context
10. Singh S, Sandhu A. Thyroid Disease And Pregnancy. *StatPearls* 21 March 2022. www.ncbi.nlm.nih.gov/books/NBK538485/

11. One in a million – the story of the Million Women Study. Oxford Population Health. 2022. www.ndph.ox.ac.uk/longer-reads/one-in-a-million-2013-the-story-of-the-million-women-study

Chapter 12: Thyrotoxicosis

1. Cancer Research UK. Thyroid cancer incidence. www.cancerresearchuk.org/health-profes-sional/cancer-statistics/statistics-by-cancer-type/thyroid-cancer#heading-Zero
2. Rahbari R, et al. Thyroid cancer gender disparity. *Future Oncol* 2010; 6(11): 1771-1779 https://pubmed.ncbi.nlm.nih.gov/21142662/
3. Abraham P, Avenell A, McGeoch, et al. Antithyroid drug regimen for treating Graves' hyperthy-roidism. *Cochrane Database Syst Rev* 2010; 2010(1): CD003420. doi: 10.1002/14651858.CD003420.pub4
4. Cojocaru M, Cojocaru IM, Silosi I. Multiple autoimmune syndrome. *Journal ListMaedica* 2010; 5(2); 132-134. PMID: 21977137
5. Orthmolecular Medicine News Service. Cancer and Vitamin C. 15 September 2010. http://orthomolecular.org/resources/omns/v06n23.shtml (Accessed 2 July 2022)
6. Orthmolecular Medicine News Service. Why vitamin C fights cancer so well. 2 July 2019. (Accessed 2 July 2022) http://orthomolecular.org/resources/omns/v15n11.shtml
7. Orthmolecular Medicine News Service. Intravenous vitamin C as cancer therapy. 14 April 2011. http://orthomolecular.org/resources/omns/v07n03.shtml (Accessed 2 July 2022)
8. Orthmolecular Medicine News Service. Intravenous vitamin C is selectively toxic to cancer cells. 22 September 2005. http://orthomolecular.org/resources/omns/v01n09.shtml
9. Robert James Graves. www.mrcophth.com/ophthalmologyhalloffame/graves.html
10. Cooke J. The Graves family in Ireland. *Dublin Historical Record* 1997; 50(1): 25-39. www.jstor.org/stable/30101157

Chapter 13: Iodine

1. Abraham GE. The Safe and Effective Implementation of Orthoiodo-supplementation In Medical Practice. *The Original Internist* March 2004: 17-36. https://tahomaclinic.com/Private/Articles2/Iodine/Abraham%202004%20-%20The%20safe%20and%20effective%20implementation%20of%20orthoiodo%20supplementation%20in%20medical%20practice.pdf
2. Gennaro AR (ed). *Remington's Science and Practice of Pharmacy* 19th edition. Mack Publishing Company; 1995.
3. Abraham GE. Iodine: the universal nutrient. *Townsend Letter for Doctors and Patients* 2005; 269. https://go.gale.com/ps/i.do?id=GALE%7CA139602813&sid=googleSchol-

ar&v=2.1&it=r&linkaccess=abs&issn=15254283&p=AONE&sw=w&userGroupName=anon~b445b84b

4. Smyth PPA. The thyroid, iodine and breast cancer. *Breast Cancer Res* 2003; 5(5): 235–238. doi: 10.1089/thy.2012.0579

5. Aceves C, Anguiano B, Delgado G. The Extrathyronine Actions of Iodine as Antioxidant, Apoptotic, and Differentiation Factor in Various Tissues. *Thyroid.* 2013; 23(8): 938–946. www.ncbi.nlm.nih.gov/pmc/articles/PMC3752513/

6. Lewis PJ. Response to Niranjan & Wright: Should we treat subclinical hypothyroidism in obese children? *BMJ Rapid Response* 12 April 2016. www.bmj.com/content/352/bmj.i941/rr-2

7. Niranjan U, Wright NP. Should we treat subclinical hypothyroidism in obese children? *Med J* 2016; 352: i941. doi: https://doi.org/10.1136/bmj.i941

8. Ghent WR, Eskin BA, Low DA, Hill LP. Iodine replacement in fibrocystic disease of the breast. *Can J Surg* 1993; 36(5): 453-460. https://pubmed.ncbi.nlm.nih.gov/8221402/

9. Abraham GE. The historical background of the Iodine Project. Iodine Study #8. www.optimox.com/iodine-study-8 (Accessed 2 July 2022)10. Redman K, Ruffman T, Fitzgerald P, Skeaff S.Iodine Deficiency and the Brain: Effects and Mechanisms. *Crit Rev Food Sci Nutr* 2016; 56(16): 2695-2713. doi: 10.1080/10408398.2014.922042.

11. Choudhry H, Nasrullah MD. Iodine consumption and cognitive performance: Confirmation of adequate consumption. *Food Sci Nutr* 2018; 6(6): 1341–1351. www.ncbi.nlm.nih.gov/pmc/articles/PMC6145226/

12. Chelson D. Your Body Needs Iodine for More than Just Your Thyroid. 11 September 2017. www.drchelson.com/single-post/2017/09/11/your-body-needs-iodine-for-more-than-just-your-thyroid (Accessed 1 July 2022)

13. Dillon RS, Hoch FL. Iodine in mitochondria and nuclei. *Biochemical Medicine* 1967; 1(3): 219-229, www.sciencedirect.com/science/article/abs/pii/0006294467900087

14. Arslanca T, et al. Body iodine status in women with postmenopausal osteoporosis. *Menopause* 2018; 25(3): 320-323. https://pubmed.ncbi.nlm.nih.gov/28953213/

15. Deville L. The iodine/estrogen connection. 6 February 2015. drlaurendeville.com www.drlaurendeville.com/articles/iodineestrogen-connection/ (Accessed 1 July 2022)

16. Korkmaz V, Ozkaya E, Cekmez Y, et al. Relationship between the body iodine status and menopausal symptoms during postmenopausal period. *Gynecol Endocrinol* 2015; 31(1): 61-64. https://pubmed.ncbi.nlm.nih.gov/25211538/ https://pubmed.ncbi.nlm.nih.gov/25211538/

17. Brownstein D. 39th Orthomolecular Medicine Today Annual International Conference. 30 April – 2 May 2010: page 52. https://issuu.com/orthomolecular/docs/omt_syllabus_2010

18. NHS. Vitamins and minerals: Iodine. www.nhs.uk/conditions/vitamins-and-minerals/iodine/ (Accessed 22 July 2022)

19. Institute of Medicine (US) Panel on Micronutrients. Dietary Reference Intakes for vitamin A,

vitamin K, arsenic, boron, chromium, copper, iodine, iron, manganese, molybdenum, nickel, silicon, vanadium and zinc. Washington (DC): National Academies Press (US); 2001. 8, Iodine. www.ncbi.nlm.nih.gov/books/NBK222323/

20. Bevan R, Nicker A (Eds). Iodine as a drinking-water disinfectant. World Health Organization; 2018. https://cdn.who.int/media/docs/default-source/wash-documents/wash-chemicals/iodine-02032018.pdf?sfvrsn=4d414c11_5

21. Eggers M. Infectious Disease Management and Control with Povidone Iodine. *Infect Dis Ther* 2019; 8(4): 581–593. www.ncbi.nlm.nih.gov/pmc/articles/PMC6856232/

22. Bigliardi PL, et al. Povidone iodine in wound healing: A review of current concepts and practices. *International Journal of Surgery* 2017; 44: 260-268. www.sciencedirect.com/science/article/pii/S1743919117305368

23. Angeles-Agdeppa I, Nacis JS, Capanzana MV, et al. Virgin coconut oil is effective in lowering C-reactive protein levels among suspect and probable cases of COVID-19. *J Funct Foods* 2021; 83: 104557 doi: 10.1016/j.jff.2021.104557

24. Handwerk B. East Africa's Oldest Modern Human Fossil Is Way Older Than Previously Thought. *Smithsonian Magazine* 12 January 2022. www.smithsonianmag.com/science-nature/east-africas-oldest-modern-human-fossil-is-way-older-than-previously-thought-180979384/ (Accessed 1 July 2022)

25. Coindet J-F. Milestones in European Thyroidology. European Thyroid Association. www.eurothyroid.com/about/met/coindet.html (Accessed 1 July 2022)

Appendix C: The PK diet

1. Bredesen DE. Reversal of cognitive decline: A novel therapeutic program. *Aging* 2014; 6(9): 707-717. www.drmyhill.co.uk/drmyhill/images/0/07/Reversal-of-Cognitive-decline-Bredesen.pdf

2. Biser JA. Really wild remedies – medicinal plant use by animals. *Zoogoer* Jan-Feb 1998. https://web.archive.org/web/20040630010109/http://nationalzoo.si.edu/Publications/Zoogoer/1998/1/reallywildremedies.cfm

Appendix E: Vitamin C

1. Drouin G, Godin J-R, Pagé B. The Genetics of Vitamin C Loss in Vertebrates. *Curr Genomics* 2011; 12(5): 371-378. www.ncbi.nlm.nih.gov/pmc/articles/PMC3145266/

2. Cathcart RF. Vitamin C, titrating to bowel tolerance, anascorbenia and acute induced scurvy. *Medical Hypotheses* 1981; 7: 1359-1376. http://vitamincfoundation.org/www.orthomed.com/titrate.htm

3. Levy TE. Vitamin C and Sepsis: The genie is now out of the bottle. *Orthomolecular Medicine News Service* 24 May 2017. http://orthomolecular.activehosted.com/index.php?action=social&-chash=44f683a84163b3523afe57c2e008bc8c.66

4. Ascorbate Web: An historical compendium of 20th-century medical and scientific literature attesting to the efficacy of ascorbate in the treatment and prevention of human and animal illnesses and diseases. 30 November 2013. http://seanet.com/~alexs/ascorbate/index.htm#Rev-Ed

Appendix F: Detoxing

1. Friedman L, Shue GM, Hove EL. Response of Rats to Thalidomide as Affected by Riboflavin or Folic Acid Deficiency. *The Journal of Nutrition* 1965; 85(3): 309–317. https://academic.oup.com/jn/article-abstract/85/3/309/4777256

2. Rea W, Md YP, Faaem ARJ do, Ross GH, Md HS, Fenyves EJ. Reduction of Chemical Sensitivity by Means of Heat Depuration, Physical Therapy and Nutritional Supplementation in a Controlled Environment. *Journal of Nutritional and Environmental Medicine* 1996; 6(2): 141-148. www.tandfonline.com/doi/abs/10.3109/13590849609001042

3. Waring RH. Report on Absorption of magnesium sulfate (Epsom salts) across the skin. The Magnesium Online Library, 10 January 2004. www.mgwater.com/transdermal.shtml

4. Pliny. *Natural History*, Vol. 9, Rackham H, transl. London: Heinemann, 1972: pp 285.

Appendix G: Diet, detox and die-off (DDD) reactions

1. Nir G. Is the sky darkest just before dawn? Davidson Institute of Science Education 9 May 2017. https://davidson.weizmann.ac.il/en/online/askexpert/sky-darkest-just-dawn (accessed 6 June 2021)

2. Fulgoni VL, Keast DR, Lieberman HR. Trends in intake and sources of caffeine in the diets of US adults: 2001-2010. *Am J Clin Nutr* 2015; 101(5): 1081-1087. doi: 10.3945/ajcn.113.080077; www.ncbi.nlm.nih.gov/pubmed/25832334

3. Cueto E. How old are caffeinated drinks? *Bustle* 16 September 2015. www.bustle.com/articles/110861-how-old-is-coffee-the-first-caffeinated-beverages-might-be-1200-years-old-so-heres-a (accessed 6 June 2021)

Glossary

1. Vera-Lastra O, Navarro AO, Domiguez MPC, et al. Two Cases of Graves' Disease Following

SARS-CoV-2 Vaccination: An Autoimmune/Inflammatory Syndrome Induced by Adjuvants. *Thyroid* 2021; 31(9): 1436-1439. doi: 10.1089/thy.2021.0142.

2. Janegova A, Janegova P, Rychly B, et al. The role of Epstein-Barr virus infection in the development of autoimmune thyroid diseases. *Endokrynologia Polska* 2015; 66(2): #39714. https://journals.viamedica.pl/endokrynologia_polska/article/view/EP.2015.0020/29453

3. Desailloud R, Hober D. Viruses and thyroiditis: an update. *Virol J* 2009; 6: 5. doi: 10.1186/1743-422X-6-5

4. Cojocaru M, Cojocaru IM, Silosi I. Multiple autoimmune syndrome. *Maedica (Bucur)* 2010; 5(2); 132-134. PMID: 21977137

5. Furab W, Kearney E, Stonny J. The presence of thyroid peroxidase antibodies in Graves' disease is predictive of disease duration and relapse rates. *Endocrine Abstracts* 2013; 31: 367. DOI: 10.1530/endoabs.31.P367 https://www.endocrine-abstracts.org/ea/0031/ea0031p367

6. Wentz I. Mold: A potential trigger of Hashimoto's. *Thyroid Pharmacist* 24 July 2019. https://thyroidpharmacist.com/articles/mold-potential-trigger-hashimotos/

Resources

General

- Dr Myhill's website – www.drmyhill.co.uk – contains 600+ pages of free useful health information. Recently fully updated.
- See also Dr Myhill's social media platforms for further support: https://drmyhill.co.uk/wiki/My_Social_Media_Presence (Facebook, Twitter, YouTube, Instagram)

Sunshine Salt

- www.salesatdrmyhill.co.uk/sunshine-salt-300-g-392-p.asp

Vitamin C , other supplements, salt pipe

- www.salesatdrmyhill.co.uk
- And numerous other good suppliers – Nature's Best, Lamberts, Viridian Nutrition, Biocare, Igennus, Now, Doctor's Best, Pure Health, Jarrow Formulas, Swanson's, Bulk (good for Vitamin C), Healthy Origins, Nature's Way.

Testing

- See 'Natural Health Worldwide' – https://naturalhealthworldwide.com/lab-tests/
- These laboratories offer thyroid function tests:
  No practitioner referral is needed for these:
  > https://medichecks.com
  > https://smartnutrition.co.uk/
  These laboratories require a practitioner referral:
  > www.gdx.net/uk
  > www.doctorsdata.com

Useful support organisation

- Thyroid UK – https://thyroiduk.org has links to private testing and other useful patient information.

Iodine supplements

- Lugol's Iodine 15% can be obtained from www.salesdrmyhill.co.uk/lugols-iodine-15-463.p.asp and https://essentialminerals.co.uk/15-lugols-iodine/ and many other suppliers.
- Lugol's Iodine 12% can be obtained from
- www.amazon.co.uk/Iodine-12-Lugols-Solution-30ml/dp/B07KTB3S7B/ and www.healthleadsuk.com/lugols-iodine-solution-12-percent.html and many other suppliers.
- Iodoral (12.5 mg) can be obtained from www.amazon.co.uk/Iodoral-12-5-mg-180-tablets/dp/B000X843VG/ and www.desertcart.co.uk/products/48162034-iodoral-12-5-mg-180-tablets and many other suppliers (e.g. www.iherb.com/uk).

Adrenal supplements

- Herbals (ashwagandha and ginseng) can be obtained from many suppliers, but for example:
  UK – www.indigo-herbs.co.uk

UK – www.hybridherbs.co.uk

USA – www.mountainroseherbs.com

- Pregnenolone can be obtained from
  Pregnenolone can be obtained from www.salesatdrmyhill.co.uk/pregnenolone-by-swansons---50-mg---60-capsules-793-p.asp and many other sources, for example:
  - https://uk.iherb.com/pr/life-extension-pregnenolone-50-mg-100-capsules/4380 - 50 mg capsule size
  - www.dolphinfitness.co.uk/en/swanson-pregnenolone-25mg-60-capsules/325050 - 25 mg capsule size
- DHEA can be obtained from:
  - Bioeva – go to www.biovea.com/uk/ and search 'DHEA' for a full list of their extensive DHEA products
  - Piping Rock– see https://gb.pipingrock.com/v2/dhea
  - Life Extension– see www.lifeextension.com/search#q=dhea&t=coveo4A2453FD
- Bovine glandulars can be obtained from:
  - www.the-natural-choice.co.uk/Adrenavive-II-Bovine-Adrenal-Cortex-Complex-150mg-90-capsules.html
  - www.dolphinfitness.co.uk/en/swanson-adrenal-glandular-60-capsules/200072

Thermometers

- FIR skin thermometer can be obtained from many suppliers, including:
  - www.amazon.co.uk/Thermometer-Femometer-Digital-Forehead-Accurate/dp/B0865RL4PH/ref=sr_1_2_sspa
  - https://lloydspharmacy.com/products/lloydspharmacy-no-contact-thermometer
- For a full range of thermometers, see www.boots.com/baby-child/nursery-furniture/thermometers

Ketone breath meters

- There are many good types – read the reviews online.
- Read this article for reviews of 10 such meters: www.msn.com/en-gb/lifestyle/rf-best-products-uk/best-ketone-breath-analyzer-for-ketosis-reviews

- Many of my Facebook Group members use this device:
  www.amazon.co.uk/dp/B07VJMNMCD/ref=as_li_ss_tl

Vitamin C urine test strips

- Readily available online. For example, see this product:
  www.amazon.co.uk/Vitamin-Strips-Urine-Analysis-VitaChek-C/dp/B00K2265JQ

NDT preparations

See Appendix B (page 117).

Index